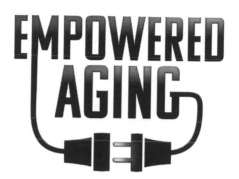

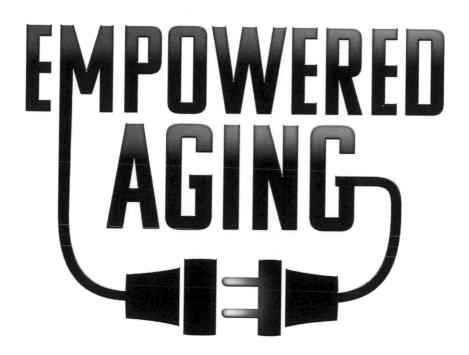

EMPOWERED AGING

Expert Advice on Staying Healthy, Vital and Active

SHARKIE ZARTMAN

with contributing
Medical, Health, and Lifestyle Experts

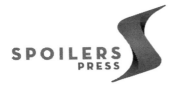

Published by Spoilers Press, Hermosa Beach, California

ISBN: 978-0-9992510-2-7 (paperback)
ISBN: 978-0-9992510-3-4 (ebook)

Book Design: AuthorSupport.com

Contents

Part 3: Integrative, Holistic and Natural Approaches to Aging

Introduction

Do you find yourself dreading your next birthday? Does it sometimes feel like your body has a mind of its own? Do you find that you can't enjoy the activities you used to love? Are you clueless about how to get your energy and your body back in shape? Do you need advice about retiring and downsizing?

Whether you are in your forties, fifties, sixties, or beyond, *Empowered Aging: Expert Advice on Staying Healthy, Vital and Active* is a collection of advice from experienced and knowledgeable practitioners about how to age successfully in a society obsessed by youth. Each chapter is written by an expert in his or her field, who takes the time to share his or her special skills in guiding others to living their lives fully regardless of age.

I created this book because I believe that the senior population deserves to have the best knowledge available to them, and as a woman in my sixties, I am not afraid to get out there and ask for advice. The idea came to me as I was talking to one of my doctors who was interested in writing a health book for the senior population but didn't have the time available. Since I love to write books, I asked him if he had the time to write one chapter, and he said yes! Then the idea hit me! Why not create a book with a collection of chapters written by experts in their respective fields on "empowered aging?" This book is that collaborative effort, and I'm so excited to share it with you.

Each chapter begins with a short author bio and picture so you can get to know all of the contributors and feel confident of their expertise. The book is divided into three sections to make the transitions easy from general topic to general topic. The first section focuses predominantly on how we can use the power of our minds and the strength of relationships to step up to aging. Reframing how we view aging, getting out and trying new adventures, building a support system and downsizing are just a few areas covered in these first four chapters. Then in the second section, we get physical and discover how important nutrition, resistance training, and cross training are for our bodies and quality of life. We also discover new medical advances for aging joints, for example: stem cell injections and platelet rich plasma injections (PRP). A life-saving, simple, and inexpensive test that detects silent heart disease is discussed along with the importance of balance training in preventing the risk of falls. Finally, the third section explores integrative medicine, bioidentical hormones, gut health, adrenal function, detoxification, and also how the brain can be kept healthy with holistic lifestyle choices. In fact, many common conditions can be treated without drugs, but rather with ancient homeopathic remedies. All of the authors not only offer you their best tips, but also write in their own voices so you will feel as though they are talking directly to you.

If you are ready to get started, open any chapter you like, take notes on what resonates with you, and start on a journey to live your best life, *now*! It's your time to *shine*!

Sharkie Zartman

PART 1

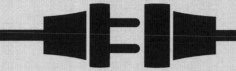

Reframing, Retirement Tips, and Downsizing for the Next Phase of Life

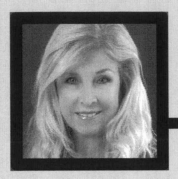

SHARKIE ZARTMAN is a former All-American volleyball athlete and champion competitor at UCLA where her jersey number was retired. She was a member of the US Women's National Volleyball Team and also competed in the Women's Professional Volleyball Association for five years and is a member of the California Beach Volleyball Hall of Fame.

As a coach, Sharkie led El Camino College to nine league and two state titles, and with her husband, Pat, she helped the South Bay Spoilers club team win multiple national titles.

Sharkie holds degrees in kinesiology and instructional technology. She teaches health and fitness at the community college and hosts "Sharkie's Pep Talk" on Healthy Life. Net Radio. Sharkie is a certified health coach with the official sanction of the New York State Education Department and the Institute of Integrative Nutrition. She is also a dynamic speaker and is passionate about inspiring people to live their best life at any age. Sharkie has authored five books, including:

- *Have Fun Getting Fit; Simple Ways to Rejuvenate Your Mind and Body*
- *Take on Aging as a Sport; The Athletic Approach to Aging*
- *Shark Sense; Getting in Touch with Your Inner Shark*
- *So You Think You Can Coach Kids?*
- *Youth Volleyball; The Guide for Coaches and Parents*

CHAPTER 1

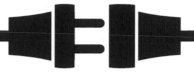

Let's Reframe Aging—It's Time to Get Empowered

By SHARKIE ZARTMAN

We've all heard the saying, "Aging is not for sissies." I never thought much about that statement because it sounded ridiculous, although now that I find myself in my mid-sixties, I wholeheartedly agree. Every living thing ages, and we humans are no exception. And as we all know, there are bound to be challenges and unpleasant changes as we get older. However, the good news is that we can control *how* we age. Don't you know people in their sixties, seventies, and beyond who are vibrant and living life to the fullest? They seem to transcend their age and maintain their quality of life. And then there are others who hit a milestone—let's say fifty years old—and decide that it's all over for them. When I turned fifty, my family *threw me an over-the-hill party*, complete with decorations, hats, and even a cake that said fifty—over the hill! I know; it was supposed to be funny, but it was the most depressing day of my life! However, it did wake me up. I have since put myself on a mission to make sure that I don't ever give up my life because of a *number*, and am passionate about helping others do the same. In fact, I want the second half of my life to be the best half. Don't you?

What do most of us want as we get older? Usually, it is quite a different list from the one we had in our earlier years. As we mature, we aren't as interested in improving our sport or looking svelte in a bathing suit anymore. Instead, we want to have mental clarity, be able to move our bodies without pain, and have enough energy to enjoy our lives to the fullest. We want to be able to play with our grandkids, travel, and make new connections. We also want to contribute to a greater cause and share our talents and experience with others. What we don't want is to feel too old to do the things we want to do, end up feeble, or be a burden on our families and society. Basically, we want to continue to enjoy our lives all the way to the end.

Is that possible? YES! However, we can't just sit back and expect these things to happen. Instead, we have to step up and take charge of our lives and habits. We are no longer coasting in life. In fact, some experts believe that most of the symptoms of aging are caused by our unhealthy habits catching up to us. So it's time to make some changes if we don't want aging to beat us up.

This chapter focuses on the mind-body connection and how important it is to get your mind on board before you do anything else. As a former world-class athlete, I know how important it is to have an empowered, *can do*, mind-set. I've seen some of the most gifted athletes in my sport elude success because they focused only on their bodies, skills, and physical conditioning and neglected their mental conditioning. However, if you spend time practicing some of the ideas in this chapter, everything can come together so that you will be so distracted by having a great life that you won't even realize that you are getting up in years. I know that if you change your mind, you can change your life. Let's explore some of the *psychosocial secrets* of *empowered aging*.

Psychosocial Secrets of Empowered Aging

What do we mean by "psychosocial secrets" of empowered aging? These are the missing ingredients in most people's quest to age successfully. Why are they considered the "missing ingredients?" Because most people don't consider them to be essential to live a vital, healthy life. But they are, and when you see how simple they are to add to your lifestyle, you will start to take charge of your health and wellness. Consider these ingredients the "spices of life."

If you have ever had a secret recipe that is both nutritious and delicious, you probably had the usual, basic ingredients that most other people have in their cupboards. But what made it special is what you added to it that others didn't.

Having a healthy, fit, disease-free body is the basic staple that we all want in our lives, especially as we get older. However, it's sometimes the little extras that make life delicious, special, and oh-so-much fun!

So here are the special psychosocial ingredients:

1. Change outdated beliefs
2. Develop a positivity practice
3. Become accountable for your choices (actions)
4. Build your own support team

5. Practice the second-half-of-life relationship rules (for us old married folks)

6. Realize that there are perks to getting older

Adding these elective "spices" to any healthy lifestyle plan will not only make it easier to get and stay healthy, it will also make life more FUN! And who out there doesn't want to have fun?

1. Change Outdated Beliefs

When elite athletes step onto a field or a court, the last thing on their minds is losing. They have a winning mind-set and most of the time are focused on what they need to do to be successful. It doesn't matter if the other team is ten times better or the odds are not in their favor. In fact, those kinds of factors usually motivate them even more.

Athletes who don't have this type of mind-set are also probably hanging onto a negative belief such as this one:

- The other team is too good. We are going to lose.
  This negative belief can be easily switched to:
- The other team is good, but it is going to feel so great to beat them or at the very least, intimidate them.

Which belief would better suit you when you step into a game? Do you think the second one would give you a better chance to win and also make the game more enjoyable? Well, we probably also have some negative, outdated beliefs (*paradigms*) about aging that could also use some rewiring.

OLD PARADIGM NEW PARADIGM

Aging sucks.	Aging is an opportunity to finally follow my purpose.
Aging is an inevitable period of decline.	Aging is a challenge and a privilege.
You stop having fun when you get old.	You stop getting old when you have fun!
I'm too old to do that.	I can do whatever I want regardless of age as long as I am healthy.
My doctor is in charge of my health.	My doctor is a part of my team. I am in charge of my health and the choices I make every day.
You can't teach an old dog new tricks.	I can learn any new tricks that I want to learn.

The old, outdated paradigms are destined to make people sad, sick, and disempowered. However, we can change our beliefs anytime we want. If you really want to make a difference in your life and your health, you have to get your mind on board.

Change your beliefs —> change your mind —> change your life.

2. Develop a Positivity Practice

"Look for the good and you will find it." This quote from the ancient Greeks is the cornerstone for living a happy, fulfilled life. The opposite is also true: "Look for the bad and you will find that too." Unfortunately, most people find themselves focused on what is wrong or what they don't have in life, complain to anyone who will listen, feel sorry for themselves, and ultimately make themselves sick. And yet, yes, I know and understand that the world in which we live now is out of control with political unrest, natural disasters, and violence. I'm not suggesting that we ignore what is going on in our world today. However, we don't need to be paralyzed by situations and events over which we have no control. So what CAN we control?

Very simply, the only things we can control are the actions we take and our attitudes.

Why is it important to practice positivity? Look no further than the mind-body connection. It is possible that our body cells may respond to our thoughts, and our physical health can either suffer or thrive as a result. We all want to be healthy in order to reach our goals and enjoy our lives, so if our thoughts are that powerful, it's time to start training our minds in the same way that we train our bodies. And the best way to do that is with a positivity practice every day.

What's a "positivity practice"? It's flipping your focus on the events in your life that normally cause stress. Did you know that your feelings are not so much influenced by what happens in your life but by how you define or perceive these events? For example, an argument can either be a depressing event or it can be an empowering opportunity depending on how you want to perceive it. We do this all the time, and once we figure out that we have the choice about how we want to view life challenges, then we can really start to change our lives.

Here is a five-point positivity plan to enjoy each and every day to the fullest:

1. Instead of asking someone, "How are you?" ask, "What's new and good?" This might stop people who were getting ready to dump their psychic trash on you dead in their tracks and force them to face their blessings and fortunes. This technique works, and it's also fun to watch people's reactions who have never had anyone ask them this question before. They sometimes look as if they are about to short circuit.

2. Practice mindfulness by trying to live most of the day in the present moment. Stay away from worrying about what might happen in the future or obsess about what happened in the past. It either hasn't happened yet—and might never happen—or it's over. And remember: Holding onto resentment is like taking poison and hoping it will kill someone else. Try to forgive and let it go.

3. At the end of the day, write down five positive things you noticed into a gratitude journal. If you do this one exercise every night before you go to bed, you will be surprised how your life changes and also how well you sleep.

4. See if you can go for a whole day without complaining about anything. If that's too hard, just try it for one hour, and then do it for longer periods of time as you start to be successful. It will be challenging at first, but keep trying until it becomes second nature.

5. Look for the good in other people and difficult situations. There's always a lesson to be learned, and every person you meet does have at least a few positive attributes. If possible, find something nice to say to a person who is upset. I find this to be a great way to get other people to shift their awareness as well. Also, it's fun to give unsolicited compliments and watch people light up.

A positivity practice not only feels good but makes you more attractive to others and affects your overall health. What do you have to lose? Remember also to be positive toward yourself and focus on your strengths instead of always noticing your weaknesses.

As John Wooden, the famous UCLA basketball coach, used to tell his athletes, "Focus on what *you can do,* not what you can't."

Each and every day is a chance to start again and fall in love with life. As far as we know, we only get one shot at this life; don't miss out by being a negative grump. Start your positivity practice today and watch your life blossom! You will also be an incredible role model for others who will want to know your secret.

3. Become Accountable for Your Choices (Actions)

This is simply taking the responsibility for your choices. You would think that this would be easy, but unfortunately, most of us have learned how to blame others for our problems. While deflecting ownership takes the pressure and humiliation off us for a short time, it also disempowers. However, once you become accountable for your actions, you finally can take charge of your life! Whatever you are not happy with in your life, see what your role was in creating the situation. Once you start practicing accountability and not projecting blame onto others, you become unstoppable! How's that for empowered aging?

4. Build Your Own Support Team

It's time to start putting together your support system otherwise known as your team. If you ever were an athlete, you most likely were chosen for a team based on your skills and previous athletic successes in your sport. But putting together a support team is different as we age because *we get to choose our own teams.* When I get frustrated with some of the people in my life, one of the best insights about understanding people comes from my husband. He reminds me to: "Limit your relationships to what you have in common." I consider this to be great advice.

Here are five tips on how to build your support team.

1. **You Must Be "All In."** In order to build a support team, you must care deeply about your quality of life and make your health a priority. Also, it's time to stop beating yourself up and realize how amazing you really are. In order be on a great team, you must be a great teammate.

2. **Evaluate Your Current Relationships.** Your family, friends, and colleagues are currently the people on your team. Cherish your supportive relationships and crowd out the negative ones by finding some new teammates.

3. **Where to Find New Teammates.** This is where we need to get bold. We are not magnets, so we must get out there and recruit, and the first place to start is in our own community. There are many community centers, senior clubs, and YMCAs that have activities for seniors including exercise classes, games, and dances. There are even some that organize travel excursions and cruises. I remember once on an Alaskan cruise, there was a vivacious group of seniors who literally "rocked the boat" with energy and fun. They made all the young couples and groups seem old. Also, there are many online communities where you can have virtual teammates!

4. **Do You Need to Fire Your Doctor?** Your medical doctors and practitioners are also members of your team, and you should be able to choose them if possible. Besides being excellent at their jobs, they also need to be people you can talk to about your concerns and who will answer your questions. Any doctor who dismisses your concerns because of your age should be fired.

5. **Be Aware of the "Psychic Vampires."** These are the people who literally complain all the time. Avoid these people if

you can because they can literally suck out your energy. I had one woman at my last presentation ask what to do about the vampire she is married to. I told her to make sure she crowds him out with lots of other people in her life who are more supportive, fun, and positive. I think I put her on a mission!

Remember, there is strength in numbers, and we need to be a part of a supportive group if we want to live an optimal life at any age. So don't be in survival mode; instead, let's be in thriving mode and be a part of an awesome team to play the toughest sport we'll ever play—the aging game.

5. The Second-Half-of-Life Relationship Rules
(For the mature, long-term, married folks)

Being married for any length of time is truly an accomplishment these days. The other day, someone asked me how long I had been married, and when I said, "Forty-two years this July," her eyes widened and she asked, "To the same person? How is that possible?"

When I married my husband, people were taking bets on how long our marriage would last. The average bet was between two weeks and two years because of our age difference and personalities. He is calm, wise, and conservative and I am the exact opposite. I did get really nervous during the vows: "For better or worse, richer or poorer, in sickness and health, till death do us part." That's a huge promise! Could I really do this?

Fast forward forty years. We are still married and happy, but it hasn't always been an easy road. Our relationship has taken many turns throughout the decades, and I'm sure more are to come as we navigate through our senior years. However, he is the father of my beautiful daughters, my lover, and always will be my best friend.

I remember someone once said, "I married you for better or worse, but not for breakfast and lunch." I never really understood that until now. Obviously, when we first got married, it was exciting, challenging, romantic, and fun! We both worked full-time, coached and played our sports. When we had our kids, the union because more challenging but was even more fulfilling. We looked forward to seeing each other when we got home to talk about our busy days. But now, as we have more time at home and our kids have moved out, we are starting to run out of things to talk about, and it seems like we keep running into each other— especially in the kitchen.

It's not bad, it's just different! So in order to keep a marriage going all the way to the end, here are six rules of engagement:

1. **Stay vibrant and interesting.** Learn something new! You can do this together or separately. No one likes to get stuck in a routine or a mundane life, so make sure you keep reinventing both yourself alone and as a couple. I see too many couples who do the same thing every day. They are bored with life and with each other.

2. **Have date nights at least once a week.** Always have something to look forward to!

3. **Make sure you don't "let yourself go."** Personal hygiene is a must in a marriage.

4. **Accept your partner for who they are.** Don't ever try to change the core or your partner.

5. **Never go to bed mad at your partner.** One of my friends said that he and his wife, when they are mad at each other, "fight naked." He said that there is no way you can fight in

bed snuggled up to someone you love. We haven't tried this yet, but if we need to, we won't count it out.

6. **Listen!** We have two ears and one mouth for a reason. We are supposed to listen more than we talk, especially in a relationship.

7. **Don't forget to say "I love you" at least once a day.**

These rules seem simple, but how many couples do you know who actually abide by them? Are these couples happy? Are they fun to be around? I saw an older couple at a restaurant the other day who sat together yet never spoke. How sad! I wanted to write down these rules of engagement on a napkin and give it to them, but I doubt they would have read it. So keep the fires burning and love the one you're with. All it takes is a little effort, ingenuity, and a lot of love.

6. The Perks of Getting Older

Okay, I get it. We are a society that idolizes youth. What could possibly be good about getting older? The terms *antiaging*, *ageless*, and *fountain of youth* have led many to believe that aging is something to be feared and somehow avoided. But the truth is, when we put another candle on our birthday cake, there is a lot to be thankful for—and no one can avoid it. Along with actively participating in keeping our health and vitality by being accountable for our lifestyle choices, it really helps to realize that there are some great perks to getting older. Seniors definitely have an edge on their younger counterparts in some areas.

Here are the "Top Ten Perks of Aging":

1. **People over fifty tend to be happier than the younger generation.** In a recent study of people aged twenty-one to ninety-nine, the results indicated that there

was a clear relationship between age and emotional health. The older the people were, the happier they felt. People in their twenties were stressed out and depressed, and the happiest people were in their nineties. The results were published in the *Journal of Clinical Psychology*. The phenomenon is referred to as "the paradox of aging."[1] How cool is this?

2. **Mindfulness becomes easier.** With all the research about how staying in the present moment benefits our health, this actually becomes easier as we age. We no longer care to think about where we will be in twenty or thirty years. We're just happy to be in the present!

3. **We no longer care what people think of us.** We can have more fun and not be concerned about looking immature or conforming to stereotypes. We already grew up, and now we can be like a kid again! If we want to paint our nails all different colors or wear clothes that don't match, so what? Live your life and forget your age.

4. **We finally have time to follow our passion.** Going to school, getting a job, having a career, nurturing relationships, and paying the bills sometimes takes up most of our energy and time when we are younger. As things start to slow down, we can finally ask, "What do I want?" Getting excited about waking up in the morning to do what you want instead of what you have to do is invigorating.

5. **We appreciate life and enjoy things we never even noticed before.** My dad always told me to "slow down and smell the bees." I thought he meant roses, but now I know what he meant. I was always too busy to notice the simple, amazing things in life like feeling the cool water and soft sand

on my feet when I walked down by the shore, or the sound of the waves, or how food actually tastes when you eat it slowly.

6. **We have life experience that is invaluable.** Most of us have been there and done that. We can become great resources for the younger generation. So what if we don't know everything about computers and technology? We know how to communicate face to face because we didn't have Google or Wikipedia at our fingertips as we were growing up. We had to learn the hard way and apply what we learned to life. We also walked to school, played outside, learned how to sew, cooked most of our meals, and made up our own games.

7. **We no longer have to raise our children.** In fact, they better be nice to us if they want any money when we move on. But if grandkids come along, we can love them, play with them, spoil them, and give them back.

8. **Seniors get great discounts!** At first, I was embarrassed to ask for a senior discount, but now it is fun, especially when they ask to see my ID first. Take advantage of cheaper prices for movies, entertainment, food, and travel. It all adds up.

9. **Self-care is now a necessity instead of a guilty pleasure.** Yes, we now need those massages, facials, manicures, body treatments, and entertainment. We need to laugh and dance and have fun. It is important for our overall health now more than ever!

10. **Each and every day is now an opportunity to love, share, experience, and be grateful.** We begin to realize that we are not going to live forever and can finally slow down and appreciate the gift of time.

Researchers and scientists are now discovering that how we *feel about our age really does matter.* If we focus on the negative aspects of aging in terms of decline or disability, our health will suffer as a result. In fact, the recent Baltimore Longitudinal Study of Aging suggests that people who are inclined to believe that older individuals are slower, unhappier and less sharp than the rest of us are more likely when they become older themselves to exhibit brain changes like those seen in those with Alzheimer's disease.[2]

How's that for motivating us to change our negative views of aging?

So are you ready to add some psychosocial spice to your life? If you can view aging as a challenge, an opportunity, and a privilege and take a proactive approach, your body will respond positively. The mind-body connection can become either your best ally or your worst enemy as you age. It really is up to you.

And the next time someone asks you your age, don't lie or be embarrassed. If you take good care of yourself, you will inspire others who are afraid of aging. Be a great role model and wear your age well. My dad is ninety-three, and he looks and acts like a vibrant man in his sixties. His motto is: "Every day above the ground can be a great day. Don't waste it!"

References

Mather, M. (2012), The emotion paradox in the aging brain. *Annals of the New York Academy of Sciences,* 1251: 33–49. doi:10.1111/j.1749-6632.2012.06471.x

Oaklander, M. "Your attitude about aging may impact how you age" TIME; Dec 7, 2015.

http://time.com/4138476/aging-alzheimers-disease/

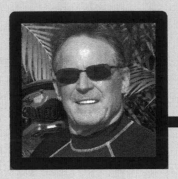

What **DON HURZELER** was: an NCAA Division Two All American sprinter/hurdler; CEO of an insurance company; president of the Society of Chartered Property and Casualty Underwriters; president of several charitable boards and foundations; columnist, author, speaker, marathoner, surfer, and family man.

What Don Hurzeler is today in retirement: wave, lava, and underwater photographer; author, publisher, beach bum, explorer, nap taker, and family man. Don is unlikely to know exactly which day of the week it is, and, yes, his calendar is open for anything fun you might want to propose.

Don Hurzeler can be reached at djhzz@aol.com.

His photographic website is donhurzeler.smugmug.com.

His author's website is www.donhurzeler.com.

CHAPTER 2

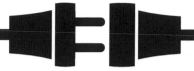

YES YOU CAN!—Don's Awesome Retirement Tips

By **DON HURZELER**

By the time you retire, you are probably sixty years old or older. You've done things the same way for a long time. You are used to the fact that there are some things you can do with ease, some you can do if you are forced to do them, and a few things you cannot do if your life depended on it. That is just the way it is. And that is the way it will continue to be for the rest of your life.

I want to call that last little bit of the preceding paragraph into question. We humans can do just about anything we set out to do. And sometimes, when we break through our own self-made barriers, there is absolute gold on the other side.

Every human being has fears—a fear of things like heights or snakes, a fear of failure or of looking bad while trying. Or, we find some things we would love to do so daunting that we just give up on even trying to do them. These are the limits we set for ourselves, and they follow us into retirement.

What happens to most of us in retirement? We center more and more on those things that bring us the most comfort and quit expanding our lives. BUT, the best part of our lives is still ahead. So, if one of your retirement gifts was a rocking chair that your friends at work chipped in to buy you, take that sucker out into the backyard and burn it! You have a lot more living to do!

I am in favor of using the retirement years to find out what is really inside ourselves. What CAN we do? Learn? Explore? And the cool thing is, in most cases, it is just a matter of deciding that we are going to move forward and try (maybe even master) something new.

A couple of reality check items. I understand that our health, physical capabilities, and finances may limit the expansion of our lives and experiences. We *are* getting older and we shouldn't be foolish about what we decide to explore. And, we need not explore new territory alone. Things go better when we find an expert or coach to guide us. Eventually, if things go as best they can, we can sometimes even become that coach.

I have a good friend—retired—whose wife always wanted to snorkel and see all the beautiful coral and fish in the ocean. Minor problem: She never learned to swim and is quite fearful of the water. The two of them came to visit. We talked about her desire to see the fish and her fears of the ocean. I told her I could take her out into water shallow enough for her to always be able to stand up with her head above water, would put floatation devices on her so she would not slip under the surface, and that my wife and I would be on each side of her as we guided her through a magical area of coral and fish. Much to my surprise—she said YES!

The next day, she got suited up, and off we went. She was NERVOUS, nervous to the point of being scared half to death. This is an elegant woman, a woman not used to looking awkward or afraid or out of her element, but off she went. She had all kinds of trouble with her face mask and snorkel. We were expecting that because ALL first timers focus their fears on that equipment— often insisting that it is such a poor fit that they cannot continue— but not our friend. She struggled through it, looked shaky, but kept moving out into the water.

Within a couple of minutes, I told her it was time to stick her face in the water and breathe through her snorkel. She did so after a few false starts with some choking and moments of panic. In five minutes, she was floating between us and pointing out fish after fish. We stayed out about a half hour and then took her past some turtles and back to the beach. A major league success! I was blown away by her guts and willingness to trust us to keep her safe. She was filled with the adrenaline of a lifelong fear overcome.

We went out again the very next day and took her into water over her head, and she did just fine. By the fifth day, we took her out to a certain point, and then had her pull her head out of the water so I could tell her this: "Sally, you are in twenty feet of water right here. If we go around this point, you will instantly be in about one hundred feet of water, and we could run into any creature in the ocean—a whale, dolphin, a tiger shark, barracuda—you name it. We know exactly how to keep you safe if we encounter any of those creatures, but we want you to know it is a possibility, and we do not want to make you uncomfortable."

She didn't even think twice about it. Her reply? "Let's go." Sally is my hero.

My wife and I decided early on that we were going to front-load our retirement with all the physically demanding things we've always wanted to do but had not done due to lack of time or opportunity, lack of funds, fear, or lack of a skill set. We decided we would save the river cruises for a much later date when our mobility was a real issue. And we got after it. I've seen my beautiful, almost seventy-year-old wife beat back really big sharks by whacking them in the head with her camera housing; cross burning-hot, active lava fields in the middle of the night to reach a crumbling cliff to photograph the lava entering into the ocean at dawn; and learn computer skills that would have been much easier to learn at age fifteen to edit photos. She was afraid of all these things but found she could do them and that she loved them. Her life has expanded more in our retirement years than at any time before.

My own personal journey has been highlighted by climbing down an eighty-foot lava cliff in the middle of the night with thirty pounds of camera gear on my back, hot, running lava all around me, and a lava delta below that could easily drop into the sea while we were on it. The lava scared me, and the climb really scared me (especially when my partner, Nick Selway, stepped on a lava tube and his leg broke through the lava tube up to his knee; the lava tube was still warm from the lava passing through it, but, thankfully, not filled with flowing 2000-degree lava). The delta scared me, and photographing CJ Kale and Nick Selway as they swam in the water right next to the lava entry scared me to death. I was quite sure one of us, or all of us, were going to die. The good news—we did not. The lesson I learned that night: I am a badass explorer and can get past my fears to do things that most people would consider, and probably rightfully, just plain stupid. But I love it.

My real test of what I was capable of doing came through my connection with a bunch of shark divers led by my buddy, Eli Martinez, the owner of *Shark Diver Magazine* and a star of his own TV series on diving with sharks. Eli proposed that we head for the border of Mexico and Belize and then go forty miles out to sea to Banco Chinchirro—a remote couple of small islands and an amazing barrier reef. The boat ride alone was enough to give me pause for thought. Eli, Linda, and I had almost bought the ranch on a similar ride a couple of years ago, when we got caught in one of those strong tropical storms that are common in that area in the summer.

I asked Eli what we would encounter once we got out there.

His reply, "Fifteen-foot-long, salt-water crocodiles in their native habitat." *Cool*, I thought. "What kind of a cage will we be in?"

His reply, "No cage; we will hold them off with our camera housings." "OK...that sounds a bit dangerous."

Eli assured me it would be safe. He may have exaggerated the safety part of the it.

Banco Chinchirro is SO remote. The accommodations are only a step up from sleeping out in the open. Phones don't work there. There is no refrigeration or electricity or drinkable water. You spear fish for your meals. You eat things like lion fish that, if prepared improperly, can kill you. Turns out they are delicious raw with a bit of chili and lemon. In all my years, I have never been in such a primitive place. The "bathroom" was a Lowe's bucket; need I say more?

Our first day there, Eli said, "Don, you're the oldest, you get to go in first." I was the oldest, alright—by about thirty years! The area we would work in was in about four or five feet of ocean water with a drop-off to the right, the island to the left, and a sand bottom with a two-foot ledge on top of which the crocodiles would come visit us—face to face. You had to keep an eye out under the boat because there were bull sharks, large Southern rays, and tarpon in the area, and crocs could sneak up on you from the darkness under the boat.

Eli told me to put on twenty pounds of lead to keep me from floating—if you float, you die—the crocs will get you. As I strapped on all that weight, I noticed that my hands were shaking, a lot. I held them up and showed them to one of my dive buddies and said, "I guess I am kind of scared."

His reply, "So am I."

I slipped into the water, and keeping my trusty camera housing in front of me, crept up on the crocs until their teeth were about three feet in front of my camera. Yes, they tried to kill us, but we had our tricks for keeping them off of us, distracting them, and had our camera housings to use as a shield if needed. When I got home I saw that my camera-housing dome had a couple of big grooves in it from the croc teeth snapping down on the dome. The adventure of a lifetime, and we all survived!

Now, I promise you, I am no braver than you are. I may be quite a bit more stupid than you, but not braver. What made me do this crazy croc thing was that I really wanted to do it, to get some great photos and to challenge a lifelong fear. Mission accomplished. Once again, I left there feeling like a badass, a pretty good feeling to have as you approach seventy years of age.

So, you have heard about my friend, and you heard about my wife, and you are probably shaking your head at the idiot that is me. I picked those stories because they are attention getters. But not all of the challenges we can take on in retirement involve overcoming traditional fear. It takes guts to try anything new— learning a new language, learning to paint, learning to author books, exploring parts of the world you have only seen in *National Geographic,* or moving from the place where you made your living to the place where you have always dreamed of living. So here are some thoughts that might be of value to you as your think about what is possible in your future...

You Deserve to See if Your Dreams CAN Come True

Dreams turn into reality by taking the actions needed to bring them into being. If you have always thought that living on a tropical island would be perfect, go live on that island for six months and see if it is everything you hoped it would be. **YOU** make your dreams come true.

Failure Is Acceptable...and Expected

It used to be so important for us to never fail. Well, in retirement, no one gives one hoot if you try and fail; it is all part of the journey. And if that island you thought was going to be perfect turns out to be filled with mosquitos and poor Internet service, you can always move again.

Abandon the Excuses

It is so easy to come up with a list of reasons not to go after your dreams. Let me start that list for you:

- You are too old to do it.
- It will be too expensive to pursue.
- It might be dangerous—terrorists are everywhere.
- You might look foolish doing it.
- Your kids and friends think it is a stupid thing to do.

There will always be an excuse to not try something -new. If you find yourself stopped by your excuses, take a look through the other end of the telescope: How CAN you make your dreams come true?

Manage the Dangers

I do some things that are way up there on the danger scale, really scary stuff with big, dangerous animals, big waves, terrain that can kill you, and in exotic locations that are in no way safe. **Here is my secret:** I surround myself with experts who know what they are doing and who are dedicated to keeping me safe. I listen to them. I do what they say. I stay hyperaware of my situation and stay calm in the face of danger. I rely on others—but I am also ready to do what I have been trained to do to keep myself safe. Is this a 100 percent formula for safety? Certainly not. But, I have noted, more of my friends have died of strokes than by being mauled by crocodiles.

My dad died at age ninety-four. He had been active his whole life. The last couple of months he was hospitalized and hated it. Two days before he died, he called me over to his bed and said, "Son, don't let yourself die like this." He then asked me how I thought I would die. I told him I would probably be eaten by a tiger shark. His reply? "Good plan...should make all the papers."

Do *not* Accept the Walls around Your Current Life

We've done what we needed to do to get to this point in our lives. We did what our parents told us to do. We did what the teachers told us to do. We followed the directions of our coaches and mentors. We did what the boss said to do. We tried to fit that all in with what our spouse or partner or kids or best friends expected of us. Cool, needed to be done. HOWEVER, we have now reached the time in our lives when we get to do what WE WANT TO DO. The only expectations that count are the expectations we have for ourselves, with due consideration with how those might fit with the expectations of our spouse or partner. **We have not reached this point in our lives to become unpaid baby sitters or day care or the transportation for whomever wants our free services.** It is our time to call the shots and make our own dreams come true. Don't let the expectations of others—even those of your beloved children—keep you from what you really want to do. You are through being told what you need to do; *do what you want to do*!

Choose Freedom

I've had every wonderful thing life has to offer. What I never had, until I retired, was the one thing that turns out to be the most valuable of all—FREEDOM. Since I never had my freedom, I really did not know what it even looked like. So I tore it apart and analyzed it. Did freedom include a job I had to be at three times a week for four hours a day? No. Did it include my sitting around the house waiting for the phone to ring for a promising consultancy? No; that is not freedom. Did it include a huge house filled with things that constantly need to be fixed or repaired? No, again. And a question for you: Does owning a pet in retirement increase your freedom or restrict it? Just a question. You will need to think differently if you want true freedom. You gain freedom with the decisions you make about how you will conduct the rest of your life.

Freedom is hard to claim, but once you have it, you will never let it go. **FREEDOM!**

And Freedom Can Be Free

My fallback position for the very small possibility that everything goes wrong and I end up penniless in my old age is the National Park system and the fabulous beaches in my home state of Hawaii. I have that "old guy" lifetime pass that cost me $10 for entrance to our National Parks for the rest of my life. Our state beaches are free to residents. I could easily be happy every day until I die visiting those parks and enjoying the ocean, rivers, mountains, and plains. You do not have to be rich to be free. Freedom is a state of mind, not a bank figure.

One Last Thing: You Are *Not* One Thing

I grew up as a corporate guy. I wore suits and sports coats. I was important. I had things to do, people to meet, goals to accomplish. I had to look good, speak carefully, and I had no time for "fun and games." I put my head down and worked. Yes, I made time for my two great kids and my wife who has now been with me for almost fifty years. Yes, I kept in touch with friends and neighbors and even tried to play an occasional round of golf. But mostly, I did business meetings, business travel, and worked. And my mind was constantly working—kind of playing a never-ending chess game that was my career and life—always trying to figure out how to survive and maybe even win in the end. And then one day, I got old and retired.

Who was I now?

At first, I was "golf guy." I played golf until my hands bled. Got down to a nine handicap, then slowly watched the handicap climb until I was a twelve and higher. The more I played, the worse I got. I gave up on the idea that I was going to get good enough to play on the Senior Tour. Golf was fun, but I wasn't good enough at it to make me feel important or admired or any of the things I used to strive for in my life. It turned out, for me, to just be a game, and that was not enough.

Next, I was "author guy." I wrote my second book. I went on dozens of TV and radio shows to promote it. The book won a gold medal for Best Career Book of the Year. I was in every newspaper, on lots of websites, all over the place. Sold a few books. Wore myself out promoting the book, and in the end, broke even at best on the book financially. I still love to write, but the reality of the publishing, promotion, and distribution end of that business is more than I want to deal with today. My future writing efforts will be low-key efforts that will be fun, take little effort, and cost me next to nothing to promote and distribute. That will be just fine with me.

And then my wife and I moved to Hawaii. I got rid of every suit except one all-purpose black suit, got rid of all the sport coats, gave away maybe fifty dress shirts and about fifty pairs of shoes. Downsized the house and our belongings. Put the Rolex away for someone to inherit down the road. Now I dress like a slob. Get up when I want to. Have no calendar to check. Cannot tell you what day of the week it is, unless the weekly cruise ship is in the harbor below our house. ("Oh, it must be Wednesday.")

I am fairly unreliable. I go out in the surf at sunup, come home to process wave photos and then to take a nap. Go out each night to shoot sunsets at the beach. Several times a week, we travel to the active lava flow to photograph it at the crater, its entry into the ocean, or somewhere in between. We travel when we want to. We just took our twelve-year-old granddaughter for a three-week trip to Europe. I have several galleries that sell the images that Linda and I manage to get.

I am not important in any way that used to count for me, but I am still important to those I love and who love me. People have no idea if I am rich or poor. As I age, I spend lots of time with dentists and doctors because I am falling apart slowly and want to do my best to stay in good operating condition. For the first time in my life, I am happy to take a back seat and let others drive or make decisions or do real work. I am very comfortable with dangerous situations and with doing things that are new to me. I do not care what others think. I am what I am and my life is what it is. My wife and I are happier than we have ever been in our lives, even though we would both like our eighteen-year-old bodies back.

That is why I say *you are not one thing*. There are people out there in the world who will accept you for yourself; they don't care who you used to be. You can survive and thrive in a new place, with an added set of diverse friends, without being a serial volunteer or the leader of the group. You can be exactly what you want to be, not an extension of who you are now. It is all up to you.

The only things that are important (aside from your faith) are these: Are you happy with your life and are you fulfilled? If you are completely happy and you've done everything that you ever wanted to do, more power to you, and I hope you keep rolling along with a smile on your face until that last moment. If not, go for a new you. *You are not just one thing.*

So, **yes you can!** You can make your dreams come true despite your advancing age. You are the one who will make it happen. If you are afraid to try, no problem, do it anyway. If you chase a dream and find that dream is not really what you thought it might be, find another. Expand your life. You deserve to have your dreams come true.

Aloha.

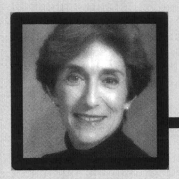

HELEN DENNIS is a nationally recognized leader on issues of aging, employment, and the "new retirement." She has been the recipient of numerous awards for her teaching at the Davis School at the University of Southern California's Andrus Gerontology Center and for her contributions to the field of aging, the community, and literary arts. Editor of two books, author of over fifty articles, frequent speaker, and weekly syndicated columnist on *Successful Aging for the Los Angeles Newspaper Group* reaching 1.6 million readers, she has assisted over 15,000 employees to prepare for the noneconomic aspects of their retirement. In her volunteer life, Helen has served as president of five nonprofit organizations and continues to serve on several boards. She is coauthor of the *Los Angeles Times* best seller *Project Renewment®: The First Retirement Model for Career Women.* Her most recent awards include the national award for excellence in educational and training from the American Society on Aging, the Status of Women award from the American Association of University Women, and recognition from PBS Next Avenue as one of the fifty influencers on aging for 2016— pushing the traditional boundaries and changing our understanding of what it means to grow older.

CHAPTER 3

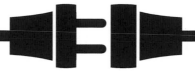

Project Renewment®: The First Retirement Model for Career Women

By **HELEN DENNIS**

This chapter introduces a new word—"renewment"—a combination of *retirement* and *renewal*. It's about career women who are passionate about their work and are facing retirement with no role models. Here's our story...

In the Beginning...

It all started in 1999 when I received a phone call from my colleague Bernice Bratter (cofounder of Project Renewment) who was about to retire as president of the Los Angeles Women's Foundation. This was her second retirement. Bernice, highly accomplished and recognized as a leader in aging, asked me, "Is there any research or programs for career women facing retirement? I'm having a difficult time."

My response in 1999 was, "No, to my knowledge there is little if any research on the subject and no programs." She further asked of my interest in the subject. Given that I was highly immersed in issues of aging and retirement, I replied, "Yes, I am interested for two reasons. One is my professional interest; the other is that you are talking about me." Although I was not then contemplating retirement, the notion of shaping the next chapter of my life was intriguing and appealing.

Subsequently, we met for a lunch that lasted four hours and realized there was a lot to discuss about issues facing women who love their work, are considering retirement, and want to figure out what is next. We then organized a dinner at Bernice's home and invited like-minded women to explore possible issues, concerns, and fears. That turned out to be a four-hour dinner.

At this first meeting of ten women, Project Renewment was born.

Project Renewment

Renewment is a word we made up as an alternative term to *retirement*. As a group, we felt uncomfortable with "retirement" since the term still conveyed negative stereotypes suggesting withdrawal, being over the hill, and not being in the mainstream. In contrast, we felt that "renewment" suggested a positive image and message about rebirth, choices, vitality, opportunity, and personal growth.

Project Renewment refers to a process that defines the dynamic changes that occur when women transform the drive and energy they previously committed to their career to another source of energy to recreate their lives. It is a redirection of focus and aspirations. Project Renewment is also a forum, a conversation group, or as a colleague described it to me, a "self-styled learning community." It also is a book entitled, *Project Renewment: The First Retirement Model for Career Women* (Scribner, 2008)[1], a *Los Angeles Times* best seller. The book contains thirty-eight essays plus a how-to guide and curriculum for forming a Project Renewment group.

From the very beginning, our group committed to focus on personal growth and to develop a body of knowledge and experience that could benefit other like-minded women. Women in this first renewment group had diverse professions: a market researcher who owned her own business for thirty years; a computer-systems analyst who did extensive expert witness work; a newly retired executive vice president of human resources; a clinical psychologist who just moved to Southern California; a newly retired women's studies and theology professor; a gerontologist specializing in aging, employment, and retirement; a business consultant; and two executive directors of nonprofit organizations.

They shared one important characteristic—not being satisfied with the status quo for themselves or their communities. Each had continued to grow throughout her career, facing new challenges and savoring accomplishments. Since this core desire for personal growth generally does not usually change with age, the concept of "renewment" seemed to come along at the right time. The group was ready to explore all possibilities in creating a meaningful next chapter of life while learning from one another and deepening an understanding of themselves and the world around them.

All of us had experience with membership organizations and raising money. Consequently, we wanted a different model.

Membership recruitment, by-laws, and fund-raising had little appeal since we had been there and done that. We fought our intuitive desire for strategic planning and goal setting. Being conscious of not getting too organized, we omitted food assignments for our next potluck dinner meeting. As a result, our dinner was colorless; it was completely white: several pasta salads, white dinner rolls, cheeses, and Krispy Kreme doughnuts for dessert. We decided that we had overcompensated for our obsessive organizational behaviors and that having food assignments was not an indication of strategic planning.

As word spread about our meetings, other professional women asked to join. Since it is difficult to sustain a group if new people continue to join, we started another group in 2001. Despite having no intention to grow, Project Renewment grew by word of mouth. Many followed the "how-to" guide that was included in the Project Renewment book about forming and launching a group. To date, we have close to forty groups that have been meeting between one and eighteen years. Actually there may be more. However, we do have a precise database of current Renewment women.

Over time, these groups have inadvertently formed small, enduring communities of highly effective, caring women who understand the concerns, complexities, and contradictions of this time of life for themselves and others. They act upon this new understanding. As one woman said, "We are approaching this next chapter of our lives in a conscious way instead of letting things just happen."

The original group now in its eighteenth year continues to meet. Some groups have ended after meeting for many years because women have moved away, died, or just dropped out. Within the United States, most of the groups are in Southern California; others are in the Boston area, Chicago, Washington, DC, Virginia, and Florida. We have a group that started in Paris and another in Reykjavík, Iceland.

A short story about the Paris group: I met with four fabulous women in Paris who wanted to start a Renewment group. After practicing my best French in describing Project Renewment, I suggested in English we have a group discussion and presented seven topics from which to choose. Among them were making the retirement decision, meaning of productivity in this life stage, the role of relationships, passion, and so on. Number seven was "sexuality." Yes, the women selected this last one. It took our American women five years to get to that topic. I said to the group, "That's the difference between American and Parisian women."

Some Rere

enewment groups have created their own names, such as "Women of Wisdom," "Women in Transition," and "the Living Group"—because they meet in a living room—and "After Labor Day"—because their first meeting was September 3, 2014, two days after Labor Day. These changes are fine with us. What is most important is to discuss issues relevant to later life that inspire women to have greater clarity about their next life chapter, and then have the opportunity to act on that clarity.

The Case for Project Renewment

For the first time in history, millions of highly effective career women are facing retirement. We are educated, skilled, and successful and have received rewards beyond money. We've made a difference and earned respect, status, and influence. We are the first and largest generation to define ourselves by our work and consequently have no established role models for retirement. According to Nan

Bauer-Maglin and Alice Radosh, coeditors of *Women Confronting Retirement*, we have a new "population of women who face retirement and are unsure of their worth without a job."[2] Clearly this does not apply to all women. Yet this uncertainty and lack of role models have served as a motivator to create a model that takes into account women's unique connection to work, their values, preferred lifestyles, ideal relationships, and what is important at this stage of life.

The market for Project Renewment is large. Among 78 million boomers, about 40 million are women; one in four graduated college and over one-third worked or continue to work in management professions and related occupations. That means about 10 million women are working or have worked in occupations that provide rewards beyond money. We also know that boomers continue to change their focus from one of success to significance, hoping to recapture their idealistic youth where one person can make a difference.[3] How to make that happen often becomes the challenge.

A Project Renewment Meeting

Typically, eight to ten women meet once a month, usually in someone's home and break bread together for lunch or dinner. Together, issues and concerns are explored that relate to retirement and postcareer living. The women who participate are proactive, nonjudgmental, and supportive. They discuss their priorities, passions, and losses to intentionally design a future that is equal to or more gratifying than their previous working years. Age ranges typically are from fifty-five to the late seventies. However, we have one group of women who are in their eighties and another group of women in their forties. Topics for a meeting usually include identity, relationships, money, health, productivity, authenticity, giving back, and more. Similar topics have been identified as important by Lisa Borrero and Tina M. Kruger in their journal article, "The Nature and Meaning of Identity in Retired Professional Women."[4]

Highlights of Four Topics

These are some examples of our group conversations.

1. Who am I without my business card?[5]

This topic deals with identity. The business card reminds us in black and white of our role and position. It tells others how to contact us and about what we do. We don't have to explain ourselves. We know that identities can become fragile when careers disappear. I recall giving a talk to a group of accountants and discussing roles in retirement. A female accountant in her later fifties got up and said, "My husband expects me to return to the kitchen and bake pecan pies and assume the full-time position of a 'domestic queen.' I hate baking and don't like pecans." Returning to a previous, full-time domestic role may not be the primary identity for many career women. Some women have created a substitute of their former business cards that reflect their new identity. Here's one: "Executive in Charge of Everything."

2. What does productivity mean, anyway?[6]

Being productive has been a mantra for many of us. It's a drive that does not necessarily disappear with age. We have adhered to the traditional meaning of "productivity" as the measurement of output and efficiency. We have fulfilled the demands and met the expectations of our bosses and organizations. What occurs when these expectations disappear and there are no performance appraisals, promotions, pay increases, or corner offices with a big picture window? What is the new definition of "productivity"? Over time, our Renewment women have shifted the meaning of being productive from believing that external circumstances must define how productive or useful we are to defining that value for ourselves. Being productive might be caring for a sick friend, doing yoga and Pilates, or having an encore career. Often defining productivity postcareer can take some time.

3. Less steam in my engine[7]

Among the grievances of our Renewment women, diminished energy ranked high, particularly for those who once had the energy of two or three people. We are talking about women who did everything—"successful on their jobs, took work home to prepare for meetings, nurtured children, applied Band-Aids to scraped knees, went to soccer games, attended children's piano recitals, entertained husband's clients, never perspired, and only fell asleep during the Adagio movements of concerts."[8] There always seemed to be a reserved tank. And then there is a change, perhaps caused by a demanding schedule or insufficient sleep. Another possible reason is age. Having a little less energy often is part of normal aging. One remedy is exercise. Research studies confirm that exercise increases energy levels, perhaps not to the level of a twenty-year-old, but that's OK with most of us.

4. What if he retires first?[9]

More couples are working today than at any other time in history. That can become a problem if our husbands are ready to retire and we are not. We know that women's work histories have often been interrupted by staying at home to raise children or relocating because their husbands have great job opportunities in other cities. Often, as women reach the peak of their careers, their husbands return home one day and say, "Honey, I just got the greatest separation package for early retirement; it's an offer I can't refuse. When can you leave your job?" Research studies indicate that retired husbands report they are least satisfied when their wives continue working.[10] For men, the most satisfying retirement is when husband and wife retire at the same time."[11] Clearly, a conversation about the retirement decision is important. Note the complexities of the retirement decision may not be an issue for many modern-day husbands. Family responsibilities often are now divided, with men taking on more nurturing roles as a stay-at-home dad, driving children to preschool, arranging play dates, or selling Girl Scout cookies at their law offices.

Here are some additional questions that have been discussed at Renewment meetings:

- The retirement decision: What are the clues?
- Is an encore career for me?
- Am I addicted to power?
- Am I antiaging or proaging or both?
- How do I prepare for "going it alone?"
- I lost my keys and my car—is it dementia?
- Who will be there for me?
- Passion is more than a fruit; how do I find the passion?
- How do I honor my wisdom?
- Forever guilty—can I read a book in the afternoon and not feel guilty?
- Play—have I forgotten how to do it?

- When to buy the plot (it always seems too early)?
- A sorority house, not a nursing home – is there a different model?

A Florida-based Group Experience

Each group's discussion is unique to its participants. Here is an example from Florida:

"We have explored many of the issues from your book and from the book, Wise Aging: Living with Joy, Resilience & Spirit, *by Rabbi Rachel Cowan and Dr. Linda Thal. Topics include: friendship, love, intimacy, meaning and purpose, children and grandchildren, mindfulness, spirituality, aging, volunteerism, and culture. As we have evolved, several of our members have had health challenges or have experienced serious health issues and/or losses with family members. We have supported one another through challenges and allowed for mutual support. We also participate in social, cultural, spiritual, and fun activities with one another. This has included visits to gardens, theater, local tours, kayaking, spa days, educational events, and the like. These are usually in addition to our monthly meetings.*

"Since the 2016 election, we have also embraced social activism together (fortunately we share similar views about the current administration). This has been an unexpected direction, but it grew out of shared concerns. We have also continued to have a very democratic approach to managing our group. We share responsibility for deciding on topics, for meeting at one another's homes, and for communication. The group has developed a level

of intimacy that enables us to share on a very deep and broad level. Most participants have expressed their surprise and delight with the intensity of relationships and the meaning that it brings to other aspects of their lives. It has been most fulfilling. This experience has enriched my life in so many ways and came at a time when my own needs found their solutions, in great part, within the context of this process."

Next Life Stages and Renewment

Renewment applies to transitions that go beyond the shift from work to retirement. After being retired for several years, women have raised different type of concerns: Should I relocate? Will I have financial security? What is my legacy? Am I living the life I want? How can I maintain my health? How does one live with the challenges of caregiving? And yet another set of questions and concerns have emerged among women in later life, some in their midseventies and eighties. Their questions have focused on spirituality, the meaning of life, death, maximizing health, living well with limitations, embracing new experiences and challenges, dealing with losses, and ways to maximize the next ten to twenty years.

Renewment is about life and change. Although the concerns and topics discussed may depend on the life stage, the format remains the same; that is, selecting meaningful topics and sharing views from multiple perspectives—historic, academic, or personal experience. The goal is to make informed decisions that lead to living a life of meaning, purpose, and dignity with opportunities to give back. Having fun is part of the mix.

The Impact of Renewment: What Difference Does It Make?

At a recent meeting of Renewment women from different groups, we asked, "What is the one thing you value most about Project Renewment?" Here are some of their responses:

"We value the continued learning, camaraderie, information, support, and learning how to make the best of my life in every possible way."

"We value the sense of caring and feeling inspired; we appreciate the challenges, the opportunities for enrichment, and having a sense of community."

"We value deeper friendships, having thought-provoking conversations, and learning about age issues."

Others have said:[12]

- "I sense opportunity for growth and exploration all around me and now am much more open to new experiences. I feel like a sponge."
- "Project Renewment has opened my mind to important issues that I now can face in a more thoughtful way than I did before."
- "Project Renewment gives content, structure, and information to this transitional period of my life. It helps to have companionship in unchartered waters."
- "I've gained just by hearing others' experiences."
- "Project Renewment has given me the opportunity to be introspective and take the time to think about reinventing and reinvesting in myself."

Here is a quick overview of the mechanics of Project Renewment.

FAQS

Q: What does it cost to be in a Renewment® Group?

A: There is no charge. Everything is done on a volunteer basis.

Q: Can I visit a group before I make a commitment to join?

A: Everything discussed in a group is confidential; therefore, typically there are no observers. One can always drop out if once you join and attend you do not wish to make a commitment to continue.

Q: From time to time, I will have a conflict that would prevent me from attending a meeting. Does that mean I should not join?

A: While we ask for a commitment to attend all the meetings, we understand that members travel and have conflicts from time to time. However, we ask members to attend as many meetings as possible.

Q: I don't like to cook. Can I bring food that I have not prepared?

A: Bringing takeout to meetings is always good.

Q: How often do groups meet?

A: The majority of groups meet once a month. Most have set times for meetings such as the first Monday of the month. Each group establishes its own calendar. Most groups meet in the evening and they have potluck dinners.

Q: What happens at a meeting?

A: Meetings often start with a check-in so members can know what is going on in each other's lives related to renewment. It is best that there is a time limit on checking-in so that there is adequate time to discuss a topic.

Q: I never heard of the word "renewment." What exactly does it mean?

A: We invented the word *renewment* by joining the word *renewal* with the word *retirement*. Retirement often is perceived as withdrawal and has associated negative stereotypes; *renewment* suggests rebirth, vitality, and opportunity.

Q: Who are the women in Project Renewment?

A: These women come from all professions. They are still working or they are recently retired attorneys, theatrical producers, newspaper journalists, market researchers, engineers, speech therapists, psychotherapists, business owners, probation officers—just to name a few.

Q: Are Renewment groups like therapy groups?

A: Renewment Groups are not therapy or traditional support groups. The purpose of those groups is to provide emotional support to alleviate a problem. A Renewment Group is most like a growth group for highly effective women. However, it is supportive.

Q: How large are the groups?

A: Most of the groups have eight to ten members.

Q: Renewment groups sound like groups during the Women's Movement. Is that movement your model?

A: Project Renewment picks up where the Women's Movement left off. Today, we have millions of career women who identify themselves by their work. They have lived before and after the Women's Movement, and they want to have their retirement years be as meaningful as their working years.

Q: I just want to hear what the other women are thinking. I am not comfortable talking in a group. Can I still join?

A: There are no observers in our groups. Everyone is an important participant. We listen, we talk, and we break bread together.

Tips for Having a Successful Group

Project Renewment members have identified the following characteristics as keys to a successful group:

1. *Authenticity*: Being true to ourselves; saying what we think, believe, and feel about issues.
2. *Commitment*: Participants attend all meetings unless they have an unavoidable conflict.
3. *Communication*: Speaking, listening, understanding, processing, and responding with clarity.
4. *Confidentiality*: Group meetings are a place where members can feel safe to be themselves and share information.
5. *Consistency:* Meetings are scheduled on a regular basis, preferably once a month on a designated day.
6. *Growth*: Groups focus on growth rather than psychotherapy.
7. *Honesty*: On an intellectual and feeling level, honesty makes the group more sensitive, aware, creative, and provocative.
8. *Ownership*: Each member is the owner of the group and takes responsibility for making the group work.
9. *Participation*: All group members take part in the discussion and no one takes the role of an observer.
10. *Personality*: Each group has its own personality to establish a successful process.
11. *Preparation*: Members typically decide on topics before each meeting.

12. *Relevancy*: Topics focus on issues most important to participants at this time of their lives.

13. *Respect*: A genuine respect for what others experience, think, believe, and envision make group discussions even richer.

14. *Responsibility*: Each participant takes responsibility for the tasks, success, and maintenance of the group.

A Final Thought...[13]

"John Gardner, in his 1965 commencement speech to graduates from the University of Southern California, addressed the subject of self-renewal and the requirements for it to occur. He said that personal renewal depends on your capacity to be versatile and adaptive and avoid being trapped in routines.

He wished the graduates something more difficult than success. He wished them meaning in life. 'Meaning is something you build into your life, starting fairly early.... You build it out of your own past, out of your affections and loyalties, out of the things you believe in...and people you love. The ingredients are there. You are the only one who can put them together into that unique patter that will be your life.'"

We embrace Gardner's philosophy. It's about renewal...at any age.

Project Renewment has evolved into a powerful communal force that reflects the drive, commitment, and awareness of career women who know that an enriching and meaningful life does not occur by remote control. There is no graduation from Project Renewment as long as we have the capacity and power to have some influence over how we live our lives. It's about the journey.

References

1. Bratter, Bernice and Dennis, Helen, Project Renewment: The First Retirement Model for Career Women. (Scribner, 2008).

2. Ibid.

3. Green, Brent. Marketing to Leading Edge Boomers (New York: Writer Advantage, 2003), p. 49.

4. Borrero, Lisa and Kruger Tina M., "The Nature and Meaning of Identity in Retired Professional Women, Journal of Women & Aging, Vol. 27, Issue 4, Feb. 3, 2015. (published on-line; retrieved October 24, 2017.)

5. Bratter, Bernice and Dennis, Helen, Project Renewment: The First Retirement Model for Career Women. (Scribner, 2008), p. 37.

6. Ibid. p. 29.

7. Ibid. p. 46.

8. Ibid., p. 46.

9. Ibid., p.109.

10. Trafford, Abbigail, "When Spouse Retired, Real Work Begins," Washington Post, October 25, 2005.

11. Moen, Jungmeen and Hofmeister, "Couples' Work/Retirement Transitions, Gender and Marital Quality," p. 55.

12. Bratter, Bernice and Dennis, Helen, Project Renewment: The First Retirement Model for Career Women. (Scribner, 2008), pp. 5-6.

13. Bratter, Bernice and Dennis, Helen, Project Renewment: The First Retirement Model for Career Women. (Scribner, 2008), pp. 13-14.

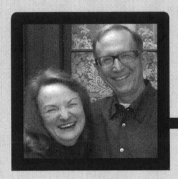

BETTY and **MIKE SPROULE**, married for forty-five years, raised two now-grown sons while pursuing careers, respectively, in marketing and college teaching. They've also traveled to forty-nine states and thirty countries. They have lived in Ohio, Texas, Indiana, Missouri, and California. Betty and Mike met at Ohio State University while on the speech and debate team, marrying after completing their graduate studies in computer science and communication.

Betty and Mike share their experiences and insights from having managed all the stuff resulting from kids, careers, cross-country moves, hobbies, and community involvement to create a downsized home that is just right for their years ahead. Their book, *The Stuff Cure: How We Lost 8,000 Pounds of Stuff for Fun, Profit, Virtue and a Better World* continues to sell in the top 10 percent of all books on Amazon.

* Sproule rhymes with "soul"—not "owl," "school," or "unruly."

CHAPTER 4

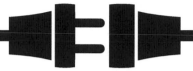

Downsizing for the Next Phase of Life

By **DRS. BETTY A.** and **J. MICHAEL SPROULE**

Everyone wants a home having just the stuff they need and filled only with things that bring joy. But how do we accomplish this? Turns out that there is no way around the need to shed holdovers that clutter the home, or worse yet, that are stored out of sight. Downsizing is not simply a matter of theoretical efficiency but rather indispensable to creating an environment with just the right stuff for our next phase of life. Pruning clutter and excess gives us the physical space and the psychological confidence necessary to embrace time and change.

While most of us easily approve downsizing *in theory*, many times we behave differently. How many long-unused items linger in your cabinets and closets, retained in hopes that, someday, they might come in handy? Also, do you hold back from giving or donating because of how much you paid for something formerly functional or fashionable, as if moving it along would represent some kind of defeat? Time and again, we refrain from pruning away almost forgotten holdovers even though they will never again contribute to our lives.

Clutter at home is not merely a problem of suboptimal storage and access. Stuff can actually entrap people, particularly as they age. University of New Mexico researcher Catherine Roster found that an excess of clutter can both physically and psychologically push persons into a dysfunctional home environment, contributing to personal distress and feelings of displacement and alienation.[1]

Common sense and academic research come together in the diagnosis that eliminating clutter will pay personal dividends. So why doesn't everybody *right now* set a goal to *un*-stuff as part of planning for the future? Well, we'll tell you why. We all know folks who have piled up possessions at home and who maybe even rent an off-site storage unit for what won't fit in their closets or garage. We may label them "collectors" or even "hoarders," yet, under whatever name, material goods keep accumulating. And at some time in our lives, these anonymous persons include *us*.

So the problem of stuff ultimately reduces itself to the question of *what to do with it*? In comments and suggestions to follow, we share a proven method to purge excess and secure our future with just the right stuff. And we want to clue you in at the outset on three especially pleasant surprises that people experience when getting rid of stuff: (1) Downsizing can be fun; (2) the effort will sometimes be profitable; and (3) the activity as a whole will give you opportunities not only to help others but also at the same time to leave the planet in better condition for future generations.

Knowing What to Keep

To overcome the heavy hand of excess stuff, it helps to begin by setting goals. At the Sproule home, we keep active in assessing and reassessing whether what we *have* is also what we *need* and *enjoy*. Coming into the crosshairs for the most severe scrutiny are things out of immediate sight resting in cabinets and closets. We equally keep in mind that prime targets must include any box or pile abiding in the garage, basement, or attic. Our metric of success comes into view when we tally boxes and count up donation receipts to find out exactly how much material has disappeared.

Early in the process of downsizing, it will help if you sort possessions by category. Why not start with clothes? Begin either with what you wear routinely or things recently worn. Apply these considerations as you take stock of casual clothing, formal attire, and work clothes. Decisions about wardrobe, or any other kind of stuff, will be easier when you work from the standpoint of criteria and categories rather than looking at each item in isolation.

Another important key to success is to begin with *easy choices*, saving the tough decisions for later in the process. Here's a tip: Don't start with things in categories holding the greatest sentimental value. Look elsewhere to begin.

Throughout the process, you will find that the *10% to 30% Rule* will become invaluable. Every time you go through your possessions, try to get rid of *one to three things out of every ten* items you review. Here we caution that if you attempt too much at one time, you'll be ever more likely to throw up your hands and give up. To illustrate, most people would experience some pain in attempting to clean out *all* vacation souvenirs at one time; similarly, trying to reorganize the garage in just *one day* probably may make you doubt whether you're really cut out for the "Stuff Cure." Even more than downsizing itself, it is the haste and overreach that actually produce uncertainty and regret. On the other hand, if you prune one to three items out of ten, you will likely feel comfortable with your progress—and over time you will begin to see BIG results.

For us, the secret of putting principles into action began with having a clear understanding of exactly what we needed to keep for the next phase of our life. From this vantage point, everything else simply became a candidate to move along. It all came together for us when we settled on three criteria for what to keep:

1. Currently Functional
2. Really Valuable
3. Outrageously Sentimental

If a particular item in our house didn't impress us with regard to at least one of these criteria, then it had to go.

What unites this trio of criteria is that all of them create an occasion to take a new look at what is in our home according to *why* we still have these things. And these criteria are not simply theoretical as will become clear in some of the following examples of how they are applied.

Currently Functional

We both enjoy a morning cup of coffee or tea. One result was that, over the years, the Sproule kitchen accumulated a stash of mugs and cups. Some matched our set of dishes, some had been souvenirs of trips and colleges, some had been promotional items, and one came in a white elephant gift exchange. Gradually, storage became an issue with around twenty mugs crammed into cabinets, some stacked inside others. And this didn't include a boxed gift set of four Christmas tree mugs stored in our garage. Helping us to keep each cup or mug was that every one came with its own story. And here we find a good illustration of how even the simplest utilitarian item might be viewed sentimentally.

So solving our problem of "too many mugs" necessitated focusing on the criterion of *actual use*. Rarely did we need more than one mug per day per person. Given that we typically ran our dishwasher every second or third day (kids long gone!), we clearly could get by with just six mugs in total. The next step was to place on the countertop all twenty-four mugs. We each picked our three favorites and put out the remaining eighteen for our next donation.

As you contemplate your own best targets for downsizing, you may be asking yourself: "But what if I might need it later?" Returning to our example, "what if we have company and need some coffee mugs we donated?" This little script seems to play in everyone's head on occasion. The best way to handle this nagging voice is to reply with a corresponding question about utility: "Have I used it in the last two years?" If the answer is no, then you have found another prime candidate to be moved along. Remember, that unless you're talking about a one-of item such as the Hope Diamond, it's likely you can replace what you've contributed to charity. When one of us needed a coffee mug for a special event, we returned to our local thrift store, this time as a customer. They had lots of great mugs for $2 each.

Now, maybe you're an artist and feel that your storehouse of materials sparks creativity. In cases where functionality meets art, it is still possible to apply the *10% to 30% Rule* to your stockpiles of hobby materials organized in that portion of the home you've defined as the studio. But remember this: While stuff sometimes inspires, the reverse is often true, too, as when oppressed by useless distractions in a cluttered space. Research by Jonathan Schooler of the University of California, Santa Barbara, shows that individuals are more creative after they have been daydreaming or letting their minds wander. In other words, stuff has very little to do with creativity. Give some thought to your own creative process and organize your artistic space and supplies in a way that have impact.[2]

Really Valuable

From our experiences in trying to sell or donate what we believed to be high-dollar items, we have come to define "really valuable" as denoting a resale accrual of at least $500. Here we are referring to *a currently obtainable value*—which would not necessarily represent the original purchase price. Even before we get to the question of depreciation, we need to remember the difference between *retail* and *wholesale*. Commonly, as soon as we take an item out of the store or box, its value to any future buyer immediately shrinks by at least 50 percent as is well known in the case of cars.

So, "$500 stuff-cure dollars" simply means an amount that someone else would be willing to pay you once they factor in depreciation, reasonable alternatives, and their position as purchaser expecting a wholesale-style discount. Periodically, we review our china, glassware, pottery, and wall hangings for sale or donation. You know something? We discovered that almost none of the fashionable items we've moved along carried a present-day value of $500 or more.

And be sure not to become confused by two seductive but essentially misleading assumptions: (1) rarity and (2) appreciation. *Rarity*? Not in the age of the Internet. Mike's dad enjoyed a retirement business as an antiques dealer during a time when local scarcities might crop up simply because no one really knew how much Weller pottery or Depression glass was actually out there. But just go online today. You'll find that what used to be rare isn't anymore! *Appreciation*? With scarcity falling like an anvil, not too many things are *ever* going to appreciate. We learned this in the case of an art print for which we paid $1500 in 1978. Present-day obtainable value? An auction house we contacted had no interest in our beautiful print at all. Why? Turns out that works by this particular artist have been cheapened by laser-print reproductions and counterfeits.

And don't be too quick to turn up your nose when someone offers you less than what you regard as top dollar for a $500-ish object. While it might seem thrifty to hold out for a better price in the indefinite future, remember that there are ongoing costs to your continuing to own an item, and these include costs of maintenance, storage expenses, and your own time spent taking care of it. And even when you've avoided offsite storage costs, keep in mind that if your stuff crowds the car out of the garage, you are encountering another kind of cost. It's a fact that the majority of Americans with a two-car garage keep one or both cars in the driveway or street.[3] Talk about depreciation!

Outrageously Sentimental

Many things that we find difficult to part with cling because we feel sentimental about them; and sentiment usually pertains chiefly to the story associated with the stuff. Strong feelings are particularly associated with items that belonged to our parents, now deceased, or were for our children, now grown. These are not just objects for us, because, when we look at them, we think of important or particularly happy times. An example of something falling into our category of "outrageously sentimental" would be the letters that Mike's father wrote to his mother before they married when he was in the Army Air Corps working on armament for the B-17 and B-29.

In our own case, most of what we cleaned out of our parents' homes when they died fell into the categories of household goods, miscellaneous artwork, and well-worn furniture. Very little of this material functionally fit with our décor, most duplicated what we already had, and little sparked the joy of memory.

But it's not uncommon for people to hold onto quite a bit of what previously was owned by dear-departed relatives because these things help us remember our family. For us, the question in this case would be of *amount*. We believe in keeping some things, but few are in a position to save everything. Betty won't forget her mother even though she's gifted or donated most of her mom's jewelry, china, glassware, and cutlery. Even a lot of the family photographs were of poor quality or duplicates. As an example of what photos to keep, Betty focused on special pictures such as one showing her mother as a young woman pictured alongside her prized horse.

Working from the other side of the generational divide, parents are prone to retain items such as a child's soccer trophy from age five. We have kept many a reminder of our days as parents, but chiefly these tokens take the form of photographs, because after our kids established themselves, we invited our sons to decide what of their old trophies or Legos they wanted to keep.

Scientists from Ohio State University have researched the

methods that help people part with their stuff. They concluded that people who take a picture of things that they found sentimental were more likely to be able to move the actual object out of the home.[4]

But again, the nagging questions crop up; for instance, "What if my children or grandchildren might want it?" Instead of just wondering about or assuming how people would react, invite your children into your downsizing project. Give them a chance to take what they want or to pick up what they think their children might especially enjoy. You may be surprised how few of your family treasures will interest your kids. We have a friend who saved all of her children's Halloween costumes thinking they would be equally wonderful for her grandchildren. Turns out the grandchildren didn't want to be a hobo, a pirate, or a gypsy. They wanted to be Spiderman, Optimus Prime, and Belle in a "real" (i.e., manufactured) costume, not something from Grandmother's basement.

"For the first time in history of the world, two generations are downsizing simultaneously," says Mary Kay Buysse, executive director of the National Association of Senior Move Managers, whose remark refers to baby boomers plus the boomers' parents. For one of her interviewees, the apparent juggernaut of home downsizing became all too real. "I have a 90-year-old parent who wants to give me stuff, or if she passes away, my siblings and I will have to clean up the house. And my siblings and I are 60 to 70, and *we're* downsizing."[5]

Little voices in one's head are particularly vexing whenever people apply the "stuff cure" to *anything* of sentiment. So this would be the point to rely on the tried-and-true principles of beginning with the easy decisions, reducing by 10 to 30%, and keeping at it.

Two Myths that Prevent an Un-Stuffed Life

You will find that the key to successful downsizing is to keep repeating: "Currently functional, really valuable, outrageously sentimental." These three metrics can become definitive for separating what is essential to your future life and what deserves to be excessed.

But even with the best of intentions to live an un-stuffed life using this mantra, there are excuses that intrude. These take the form of tales we tell ourselves and that introduce barriers stemming from nagging regret or lingering guilt. Here are the most common ones that we hear.

"I don't have a problem, but my husband/wife is a packrat." Someone else's precious stuff often looks like junk to others. We advise keeping mum about other people's things, and instead, setting an example by first downsizing your own stuff. If your objective alternately requires engaging your partner in downsizing, begin to work as a team with a focus on the future as you try to find the wins in creating your future environment together and at the same time perhaps sparking joy in others who may benefit from your excess.

"Off-site storage can solve the problem." Let's begin with the truism that there probably isn't anything that we would call *currently functional* in your storage unit simply because of limited access. With respect to value and sentiment, try to reframe your unit as an un-stuffing staging area from which you would gradually transform unused materials into gifts or donations if these are items that you wouldn't want to bring back home. If you wanted to operate on a grander scale, you might arrange for a charitable organization to bring a truck to meet you at your storage unit; anything too broken down or unusable would be prime for recycling or the dump. Won't you enjoy no longer paying that monthly bill from the storage company?

And we can also learn from the case of Fred and Claudia who, having a chance to move to Italy for Fred's work, rented their home unfurnished and stored their household goods and keepsakes offsite. Months turned into years, and soon their storage fees of $100/month totaled more than $13,000. Returning home, they hired movers to pick up their furniture. As the men unloaded the truck, Fred and Claudia found that their goods looked more like "bads"—an assemblage clearly more miscellaneous, worn, and out of style than they remembered. Some of it was not only dusty but a bit moldy.

The "Seven Morphs"—Changes to Your Behavior

No matter how successful we are at a one-time downsizing of rooms, closets, basements, attics, and garages, the un-stuffed life will remain out of reach unless we keep up the effort. What this means is that we must change some old behaviors to keep the excess from piling up in the future.

We affectionately call these changes the *Seven Morphs* to help us remember that ongoing change is essentially a commitment to always living with just the right stuff. Especially after your sixtieth birthday, it's high time to embrace the seven morphs and whistle while you work.

1. Refraining. The more you get rid of stuff, the more you will recognize that everything has to move along at some point. But the most fundamental way to un-stuff your life is to never acquire the things in the first place. "Stuff avoidance" pertains especially to things that are free, such as informational brochures, water bottles, T-shirts, and coffee mugs. Why not recycle at the source by not accepting some of the advertising-related goods offered to you? You can also switch more of your routine bills and correspondence to electronic communication so you don't have as much paper to file and then shred.

2. Restraining. Sometimes, when you can't say "no," you can say, "just a little." This way, you can still buy the things that you want, but you don't have to buy in bulk right now. Especially when you're shopping locally where you can easily return for more, start with only the immediately necessary quantity and then add more if you really like what you have tried or need or want more. Many people who shop at big box stores find their shopping carts overflowing because they think they are getting a bargain. But in cases such as paper products, the savings may be very small, especially when considered against the inconvenience of cramming them in the basement or garage.

The *theory of displacement* can come in handy at this point. When you get something new, get rid of something old; this principle served us well with respect to some new towels. A variation would be to begin depleting inventories. Too many bottles of wine? Why not invite friends over to share? Why not give away some of your prime vintages?

3. Returning. Everyone has experienced buyers' regret, and who among us has not received a gift that will *never* keep on giving? Here the key is to move quickly. Return your purchase to the store for a credit while the object is still intact and you can find the receipt. While this sounds like an obvious suggestion, it's not uncommon for people to donate clothing that comes complete with original tags. The National Retail Federation reports that one-third of all gifts are returned or exchanged, so know that you are not alone in occasionally returning an item.[6]

4. Reusing. We encourage people to donate to local charity thrift shops and also to shop at these same stores. In fact, think of your local thrift shop as your storage unit. In this scenario, you bring them the stuff that you are not currently using. If you ever need the same or an equivalent item, you'll find it waiting for you all cleaned up and ready for purchase at a reasonable price.

5. Renting. The Internet has made renting and shared use so much easier to manage. Renting and group buying allow us to solve the problem of un-stuffing before we ever acquire the stuff. Rent the roll-away bed on the rare occasions that your house is filled up with guests. Purchase a chainsaw with a neighbor. When you get more use out of existing stuff, you benefit the planet at the same time that your life becomes easier and less costly.

6. Recycling. Options for recycling unused stuff vary greatly by locality, so check options at your local waste management website. Paper seems particularly prone to mounting up as clutter, and fortunately, most of this can be recycled. Shredded white paper and aluminum cans are particularly desired at recycling centers. In our case, we live in a city where recycling is free and trash requires a fee for pick-up—a powerful incentive.

7. Rendering into Trash. We've all seen things placed at the curb that seem to be in better condition than something we are currently using in our house! Try not to take the lazy way out by using the trash can as your go-to place for downsizing. Of course, if it's broken or filthy, trash it. Remember to be responsible and consult your local waste management office for places to get rid of fluorescent bulbs, batteries, paint cans, and the like.

Tips for Success and Fun

As we talk to people about their experiences in getting rid of excess stuff, they typically report having viewed downsizing as a chore to be endured. Yet once you get the hang of it, you may find that un-stuffing becomes something like a hobby or a mission, bringing feelings of satisfaction and pride of accomplishment. Consider these ways to change your attitude toward downsizing.

Give yourself permission to get rid of stuff. After saying you'll clean out your closets someday, seize the day. Some people are forced to downsize because of a tragedy or financial hardship. So if you're in a position to downsize by choice and at leisure, count yourself lucky. And don't feel as if you have to go it alone. Involve your family; everyone will enjoy the improved environment. And maybe inject a bit of friendly competition in making a charitable donation or preparing for a garage sale. If you know people who would like what you are moving along, invite them over. Ask for tips about where to donate from people you know who like to shop at thrift stores.

Create a replacement budget. A win-win strategy for planning ahead and for motivating un-stuffing is to keep records of income from sales of stuff together with estimates of money you saved by retiring the rented storage space or from deductions on your taxes. Don't forget to estimate the value of the space that you have freed up in your home by multiplying square footage times the typical sales price per cubic foot of real estate in your area. Then there's the weight-watchers aspect: keep track of the volume and/or weight of the stuff that you are moving along. Money from sales, exchanges with friends, and tax deductions can be used as a rainy-day fund on those *rare* occasions that you need to buy something very much like what you got rid of.

Create an un-stuffing staging area. We've already mentioned using your storage unit as a jumping-off point for downsizing. This principle applies to your home as well. Find a space—or maybe more than one—where you can place things you believe might be un-stuffed, for instance, a shelf box in the closet or a bag in the basement. After items have stayed in the staging area for a couple of weeks, you will find that they tend either to migrate back into a pattern of active use or that your resolve increases to package them up for donation. If you itemize deductions on your income taxes, you can donate up to $250 in any one drop-off with just a receipt and with no appraisal.

Realize that downsizing does take effort. In a consumer society, choosing to live without excess stuff requires affirmative and sustained effort. If you would like help, you can hire a professional to accelerate your progress by consulting local members of the National Association of Senior Move Managers at www.nasmm. org or the National Association of Professional Organizers at www. NAPO.net.

If you've been motivated to read to the end of this chapter on downsizing, it's a sign that you are ready to take a serious stab at the Stuff-Cure! Let's get started!

References

Roster, Catherine & R. Ferrari, Joseph & Jurkat, Martin. (2016). The dark side of home: Assessing possession 'clutter' on subjective well-being. *Journal of Environmental Psychology*. October 10, 20164. https://www.researchgate. net/publication/298428874_The_dark_side_of_home_Assessing_ possession_%27clutter%27_on_subjective_well-being

Jonathan Smallwood and Jonathan W. Schooler. (2015). The Science of Mind Wandering: Empirically Navigating the Stream of Consciousness. *Annual*

Review of Psychology 2015 66:1, 487-518. http://www.annualreviews.org/doi/abs/10.1146/annurev-psych-010814-015331

Emma Johnson. The Real Cost of your Shopping Habits. *Forbes.* January 15, 2015. https://www.forbes.com/sites/emmajohnson/2015/01/15/the-real-cost-of-your-shopping-habits/#edb3e031452d

Karen Page Winterich, Rebecca Walker Reczek, and Julie R. Irwin (2017) Keeping the Memory but Not the Possession: Memory Preservation Mitigates Identity Loss from Product Disposition. *Journal of Marketing*, Volume 81, Issue 5 September 2017. http://journals.ama.org/doi/abs/10.1509/jm.16.0311?code=amma-sitehttp://journals.ama.org/toc/jmkg/81/5

Richard Eisenberg. Sorry, Nobody Wants Your Parents' Stuff. *Forbes*, February 12, 2017. https://www.forbes.com/sites/nextavenue/2017/02/12/sorry-nobody-wants-your-parents-stuff/#5c6b4dc924ed

National Retail Federation. *2015 Consumer Returns in the Retail Industry.* © December, 2015 The Retail Equation, Inc. https://nrf.com/sites/default/files/Images/Media%20Center/NRF%20Retail%20Return%20Fraud%20Final_0.pdf

PART 2

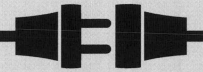

The Care of the Body: Nutrition, Muscles, Joints, the Heart, and Balance

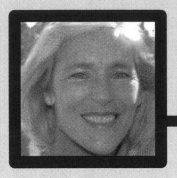

JEANNE PETERS, RD, Nutrition Director of the Nourishing Wellness Medical Center, is on a mission to help people of all ages develop healthy, lifelong eating habits that contribute to greater health and well-being. In the past twenty-eight years, she has followed a career path that has earned her recognition as an expert in food and nutrition education. She received her BS degree in Clinical Nutrition from the State University of New York at Buffalo. She is the former nutritionist for the LA Kings hockey team, designed the Deal-A-Meal program for Richard Simmons, and developed a nationwide preventative health program for Pritikin Systems, Inc. and fitness guru Kathy Smith. She has also created healthy food programs for Bristol Farms, Inc., Mattel Corp., Quaker Oats, and Chevron. Recently featured as nutritionist for Discovery Channel's *Fit TV Ultimate Goals* series and sought-after nutrition expert, she is the author and radio cohost of the weekly show *Nourishing Wellness.* Named California Young Dietitian of the Year in 1995, she specializes in hormonal balance and weight management with her husband, Dr. Allen Peters, at their medical office in Torrance, CA.

CHAPTER 5

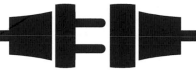

The Food Rx to Reverse Aging

By **JEANNE PETERS, RD**

Mark Twain once said, "Life would be infinitely happier if we could only be born at the age of eighty and gradually approach eighteen"; however, there are numerous studies that indicate we can slow down and even reverse the aging process through measurable improvements of the key biomarkers or critical tests that determine how fast or slow you are aging.

As a registered dietitian (RD), I work in tandem with my husband, a holistic medicine doctor in our practice at the Nourishing Wellness Medical Center, where we specialize in age management medicine—the science of helping men and women in midlife extend their health span and longevity. We not only look at the physiological (physical) external effects of aging, such as wrinkles, hair loss, and weight changes, but also internal changes: hormone imbalance, thinning bones, failing memory, rising inflammation, and declining mood. These are very real challenges that prevent us from feeling and looking our very best; however, we believe there are critical food and lifestyle choices that can reverse aging at the cellular level and lower the risk of age-related illnesses.

The 90/10 Rule

In fact, science has proven that 10 percent of aging is caused by genes, while 90 percent is caused by environmental factors, including lifestyle choices. I call this the 90/10 rule: Genetics loads the gun, and the environment pulls the trigger. Therefore, we teach our patients how to upgrade their food and lifestyle practices in order to overcome this genetic 10 percent. Our fifty- to eighty-plus-year-old patients have taught us that it is never too late or too early to slow the aging clock with better food and lifestyle choices.

Want to know more about our "food first" philosophy that we teach our clients? It's based upon the science of *nutrigenomics,* or how food communicates with your genes. We know that the quality of your food determines which genes turn off or turn on to improve your health. For example, Dr. Dean Ornish, MD showed that after just three months on an intensive lifestyle program, including a whole-foods, plant-based diet, over five hundred genes that regulate cancer were beneficially affected, either turning off the cancer-causing genes or turning on the cancer-protective genes.[1] No medication can do that! Remember with every bite you eat, it's a chance to heal your body. Food is your best medicine. What you put on the end of your fork is more powerful than anything you'll ever find at the bottom of a pill bottle.

Let's discover the food-related issues that can accelerate the aging process, and conversely, how adding in more nutrient-dense, antioxidant-rich, real foods can help you look and feel better so you can enjoy more life in your years ahead.

Issues that Accelerate the Aging Process

There are many issues and theories that have been identified with accelerating chronic disease and the aging process. Some of these include: chronic stress; lack of deep sleep and regular exercise; toxic exposure; oxidative damage from excessive free radical damage to the mitochondria, which are the energy-producing cells of the body; chronic inflammation; and poor blood-sugar control. Let's examine in more depth three of these issues that accelerate aging.

Free Radicals, Oxidation, and Mitochondria

Many longevity researchers agree that free radicals are the main culprit in damaging our bodies as we age. They cause cells to degenerate by means of a chemical process known as *oxidation*. Besides damaging cells and organs, free radicals adversely affect the *mitochondria*—the powerhouse of each cell that provides the energy needed to sustain life. Mitochondria are different from other cells in that they contain their own DNA. The old saying that "there's no such thing as a free lunch" applies to the energy production by the mitochondria. When energy is produced inside the mitochondrial membrane, *free radicals* and hydrogen peroxide are produced. These radicals can inflict considerable damage to the cellular structure of the mitochondria as well as to the mitochondria's DNA. Antioxidants found naturally in fresh, colorful plant foods can help the body repair the damage to cells caused by free radicals. [2]

Inflammation. *Inflammation* is a normal and beneficial process that occurs when your body's white blood cells release chemicals to protect affected tissues from foreign invaders like bacteria and viruses. The release of these chemicals increases the blood flow to the area of injury or infection, and may result in redness, warmth and swelling. This is classic acute inflammation.

You actually need some level of acute inflammation in your body to stay healthy; however, it's increasingly common for the inflammatory response to get out of hand and become a chronic issue. This process can go on for years without symptoms, often silently damaging your tissues without notice until there is a loss of function, such as bad joints, or a disease develops, for example, asthma, allergies, autoimmune disease, heart disease, or cancer. We are seeing an epidemic of inflammatory diseases that affect 125 million Americans. That means in the average family of three, at least one person has a chronic disease caused by inflammation. [3,4]

In our practice, we do food sensitivity testing on anyone with lab tests and signs of chronic inflammation. What foods are the biggest culprits of inflammation? Continue reading.

The Seven Sinister Foods of Inflammation

The seven sinister foods that increase inflammation include the following:

1. gluten (wheat, barley, rye, oats, spelt, kamut)
2. dairy (milk, cheese, yogurt),
3. corn
4. eggs

5. soy

6. nuts/seeds (peanuts, cashews, almonds)

7. nightshades (this includes a group of plants such as tomatoes, bell peppers, chili peppers, potatoes, eggplant, cucumbers)

These foods can also cause acute allergic and inflammatory reactions. But these are rare and generally affect less than 1 percent of the population. For more than 50 percent of us, however, these seven foods prevent us from living a vital, healthy life.

Dairy and gluten are the most common triggers of food issues linked to insulin resistance. They worsen damage by making you hungry for more food. Taking them out of the diet allows the inflamed gut and an inflamed body to heal.

Sugar and Toxic Fats

Two other inflammatory foods include sugar and toxic fats.

Sugar: Want to jump on the fast track to reverse aging? Yes, you do! Aim to greatly reduce or eliminate sugar and sugar substitutes! This includes: white table sugar, agave, brown sugar, sucralose (Splenda), aspartame, maple syrup, and molasses. Stay away from hidden sugars in ketchup, salad dressings, sauces, and packaged cereals. If sugar is one of the first six ingredients, avoid it.

Foods high in sugar are addictive because they trigger the reward centers of your brain. While sugar triggers the release of *dopamine*, the brain chemical of pleasure, satisfaction, and reward, sugar also harms the *hippocampus*, the part of the brain responsible for memory and the regulation of emotions. While it's not perfect, the *glycemic index* rates carbohydrates based on how they affect blood sugar, and *all* sweeteners take blood sugar levels for a roller-coaster ride—they spike and then plummet. There are a few sweeteners that don't spike blood sugars and are acceptable, like stevia, lucuma powder, and monk fruit.

Toxic Fats: Refined oils are often processed with chemicals and harsh solvents, or they're hydrogenated which means that high heat is applied to liquid oils along with which then creates toxic fats, called trans fats. Think of the way French fries are made. These toxic fats increase inflammation in the body. Aim to avoid the industrial oils such as canola, corn, cottonseed, vegetable, soybean, and sunflower. In order to produce these oils, often there are chemicals used to extract the fats from the seed or grain. This processing of industrial seed oils are linked to higher rates of inflammation and problems with insulin and blood sugar regulation.

Instead, focus on using the following type of fats for cooking or salad dressings: Cold pressed avocado or olive oil, butter, ghee-which is a dairy free butter or cold pressed coconut oil.

What Is the Connection between Insulin, Blood Sugar, and the Aging Process?

The level of *insulin sensitivity* of the cell is one of the most important indicators of how long a person will live (or, as we say in the medical profession, a "marker of lifespan"). Here is how it works.

The main job of insulin is to regulate your blood sugar. The more sugar you consume, the higher the amount of insulin is needed to deliver glucose as fuel to your cells. Think of insulin as the knock on the door to your muscle, liver, and fat cells, announcing, "Here comes sugar, whether you need it or not!" Those cells will politely receive insulin's invitation and allow glucose in. With this supply of glucose, your cells can tackle important tasks such as muscle growth, movement, and repair. All is fine until your cells become so full of sugar that they can't absorb any more (just like a sponge). [5,6]

At this point, they stop listening to insulin. They've had enough sugar! But insulin won't take no for an answer, so it knocks louder and louder. After every type of cell puts up a "keep out" sign, one type of cell usually responds to insulin's call: *your fat cells.* Fat cells will remain "best friends" with insulin, and most of this fat accumulates in places like your belly, hips, and thighs. If you consume a diet consistently high in sugar and grains, over time your body becomes "sensitized" to insulin and requires more and more of it to get the job done. Eventually, you become "insulin resistant," which increases your risk for diabetes.

The way out of this conundrum is to reset your insulin level by reducing and even eliminating highly processed, starchy carb's from grains like wheat, corn, and soy based foods like crackers, cereals, baked goods, and pasta in your diet. You'll be amazed at the big improvement in your blood sugar levels with this one technique.

Through our food choices, we can switch our body from being a "sugar burner" to a better "fat burner." Let's look at how to make that switch by examining which foods are best to eat.

What Should You Eat?

We advocate a "low inflammatory diet." This means moderate protein, moderate fat, minimal sugar, lots of greens and other vegetables balanced with one to two servings of low-sugar fruits. Start with replacing some of the processed, packaged foods you consume with more fresh, nutrient-dense foods that grow in the ground. The steps listed below will help you make this transition. And the best part is

that you can find most of the tools and foods you need to age well...
at the grocery store. Let's get started!

Eat LEAN PROTEIN at Every Meal

Protein is a key macronutrient to help repair your body. It forms the
building blocks of your lean muscle mass and feel-good, energizing
brain chemicals. Protein at every meal is analogous to adding a well-
seasoned log on a fire—it provides steady energy to keep your blood
sugar stable for a few hours. It also boosts your immune system and
builds a strong fortress in your gut. Aim to include some lean animal
or plant protein sources at every meal.

Best Choices: Choose free-range, cage-free, grass-fed, and
no-hormone-added sources whenever possible. For fish, aim for wild
caught. Some examples include: lean chicken and turkey, eggs, cold
water fish (sardines, salmon, cod, trout, mackerel, tuna), shellfish,
bison, lamb, wild game, whey protein, tempeh, and lentils.

Eating Tip: Aim to eat at least half of your ideal body weight
in grams of protein each day. For example: A 150 lb. person would
consume about 75 grams of protein a day divided among a few
meals. For example, you would eat 15-21 grams per meal or snack.
This is equivalent to about two to four ounces of plant-based or anti-
inflammatory animal protein at each meal, which will help activate
your longevity genes. Ideally, your protein intake will make up about
15-20 percent of your daily calorie intake.

Eat Beneficial Fat at Every Meal

Fat is a vital nutrient that your body needs for a wide range of
biological processes, including growth, healthy skin, and for
absorbing nutrients. It's also an important fuel source. Eating the

right fats, in moderation, will help you feel full faster, and in turn, decrease your appetite and cravings between meals. They can even help lower your risk of heart disease by reducing your levels of total and LDL («bad») cholesterol. Many fats like fish oils offer anti-inflammatory benefits and are useful to supplement to get the essential omega-3 fats, DHA and EPA, which help lubricate the tissues of your eyes, brain, blood vessels, joints, and more.

Best Choices: Choose cold-pressed extra virgin coconut, olive, or avocado oil. For cooking at medium high heat, use coconut oil, red palm oil, butter, and other saturated fats such as tallow (beef fat) because they do not get oxidized like olive oil does. Only use olive oil for low-heat cooking. Beneficial whole food fats include avocados; nuts like pecans, macadamia, hazelnuts, and walnuts, plus nut butters; seeds; olives; and coconuts. **Medium-chain triglyceride (MCT) oil** is a very efficient type of oil derived from coconuts that rapidly converts into energy for your brain and body and doesn't require a stop at the liver for processing. (You don't need bile acids to digest it.) Use MCT oil (these letters mean medium chain triglycerides found in coconut oil) or salad dressings and drizzling on steamed vegetables. **MCT oil can be found in the supplement section of a natural foods store or online.**

Eating Tip: Aim to get a serving at every meal and snack for satiety. At least 45-50 percent of your daily calories can come from healthy fat sources. For example, if you need 2000 calories to maintain your current weight, at least 1000 calories can come from fat sources. Use a food tracking app like MyFitnessPal.com to determine what percentage of your total calories are coming from fat. Studies show that when people trade processed carb calories for fat, they have better long-term dieting success because they feel a greater sense of fullness between meals and reduce their total calorie intake all the while feeling less hungry and having fewer cravings.

Enjoy Colorful Carbohydrates at Every Meal

Most of your carbohydrates each day should come from real food sources such as vegetables, a couple of fruit servings, and a small amount of starchier carbs like sweet potatoes to balance out your calorie needs. A benefit of eating this way is that these foods contain large amounts of fiber, which increase *satiety* (your sense of fullness and sense of meal satisfaction along with the many colorful antioxidants and phytochemicals, which are the natural plant chemicals that fight all diseases. This is a winning combo for your health goals!

BEST CHOICES

Vegetables. Enjoy a rainbow of color on your plate! Getting a wide variety of color in different kinds of produce ensures that you're getting the thousands of phytochemicals that science has shown reverse the aging process. Of all the plant colors, research shows that green foods have marked beneficial effects on cholesterol, blood pressure, immune response, and cancer prevention. These effects are attributed in part to their high concentrations of **chlorophyll.** So enjoy plenty of deep greens like arugula, spinach, swiss chard, parsley, and all herbs. Finally, try some cultured vegetables like kimchi and raw sauerkraut, too. These vegetables provide lots of natural enzymes that improve digestion of proteins, plus they offer millions of probiotics that support a healthy GI and immune system.

Fruits. Eat fresh, whole fruits instead of drinking juice. Fruits vary widely in the amount of sugar and fiber they contain. For example, most of the tropical fruits like mango, papaya, pineapple, and melons naturally contain more sugars, so enjoy your portion after a hard workout where the sugars will be burned quickly. All berries are your best bet for daily consumption. They put the least amount of sugar in your blood and contain some of the highest levels of antioxidants of all foods. Blueberries also increase brain power and improve memory. You'll get the same health benefits if you eat them fresh or frozen; a good choice is wild organic blueberries found in the freezer section of most supermarkets.

Starchy Carbs. Trade the "white stuff" like flour, sugar, pasta, bread, and processed baked goods for more calorically dense but wholesome choices like millet, sorghum, beets, yams, turnips, parsnips, and squash. These foods contain more than twice the amount of calories per bite as most of the vegetables that grow above the ground, so be mindful of your portion size to meet your calorie needs.

Eating Tip: Aim for 4-5 cups per day. One rule of thumb to increase your fruit and vegetable intake is to add one serving to each meal. For example, **make a vegetable or fruit smoothie!** This is an awesome way to max out your intake for the day for a morning on the run or for a post-workout snack. (See the meal ideas at the end of this chapter.)

Include raw, cooked, and even vegetable juices for variety. This habit will transform your energy levels through the additional phytonutrients and antioxidants needed to squelch the free radicals we produce all day long.

After a hard exercise session, reward your body with a serving of starchier carbohydrates or a full portion of fruit and consume within an hour of exercise. They are burned more efficiently after exercise instead of being stored as belly fat.

What Beverages Are Best?

Drink More Water. Drink healthy, nondistilled, pure filtered water each day. How much? Divide your ideal weight in half, and then drink that amount of water in ounces each day. For example, a woman weighing 120 pounds would need to drink 60 ounces, or about 7.5 cups a day. To increase hydration from water, add a tiny pinch of sea salt or a squeeze of fresh lemon or lime to each glass. Doing so helps alkalize the water, which will enable the water to be carried more efficiently into the cells, thus improving the cells' ability to flush out toxins.

Enjoy a Cup of Coffee. Coffee is the biggest source of antioxidants in Americans' diets, and more than half of the people in the United States drink coffee every day. Two 2017 studies published in the *Annals of Internal Medicine* correlate coffee drinking with a longer lifespan. A large European study found those participants who drank the most coffee had a 10 percent lower risk of dying from any cause compared to those who didn't drink any coffee at all. But your java can be tricky when it comes to your genes—some people are genetically tuned to metabolize the caffeine better than others. Those who struggle to digest it (feeling wired or jittery are common signs) would benefit from keeping it to one cup a day or swapping it for decaf or organic green tea; otherwise, it could be taking its toll on your sleep. [7,8,9]

Take a Tea Break. Both green tea and Tulsi tea contain compounds known as *polyphenols,* which help to eliminate inflammation-producing free radicals. Recently, researchers have found that these polyphenols protect healthy cells from cancer-causing DNA damage while ushering cancer cells to their death. Another remarkable finding is the power of green tea polyphenols, known as EGCG, to reactivate dying skin cells. This means your skin can regenerate and your wrinkles will lessen over time by simply enjoying a few cups of green tea daily.

Alcohol. When it comes to alcohol, try to stick to red wine. It contains a substance called resveratrol that helps your body fight off age-related illnesses. One glass of organic red wine three to four times per week delivers optimal health benefits—studies have shown red wine can reduce an early death by more than 30 percent. Be wary of exceeding four glasses per week, however, as this will put unnecessary strain on the liver. As we age, our liver struggles to do its job; if you're keeping it busy with alcohol, this explains why hangovers hit harder with age.

Some Suggestions for Low-Inflammatory Meals

BREAKFAST

1. 2-3 sunny-side-up eggs +1 cup cooked spinach, tomato, bell peppers, mushrooms +1/2 avocado + 1/3 cup of fresh berries + water with fresh lemon or pinch of sea salt.

2. ½ cup egg or chicken salad wrapped in large leaves of lettuce for a quick breakfast wrap.

3. **Brain-Boosting Smoothie:** 1 scoop egg, whey protein, or collagen powder, 1 cup unsweetened almond or coconut milk, 1/3 fresh wild blueberries, 1 tbsp. of psyllium flakes,1 tsp of cinnamon, 1 tbsp of MCT oil or coconut oil.

LUNCH/DINNER

1. ½ cup egg or chicken salad wrapped in large leaves of lettuce for a quick veggie wrap + iced green tea.

2. 3-4 oz grilled breast of chicken, sliced over 3 cups of mixed

deep colored greens, canned artichokes, grated carrots, black olives + 2 tbsp of lemon juice with 1-2 tablespoons of olive oil.

3. 3-4 oz broiled wild caught salmon, grass-fed steak or lamb, 1 cup steamed asparagus with a 1 tsp of melted butter and fresh lemon + small baked yam + glass of red wine.

HEALTHY SNACKS

1. 1 12 oz bottle of Evolution Green Juice with lime or other low-sugar, greens-only juice + ¼ cup of dry roasted almonds or macadamia nuts.

2. 1 tbsp almond butter + ½ apple, thinly sliced.

3. 10 black olives + 4 stalks of celery.

4. 2 hard-boiled eggs + dab of mustard or pesto + fresh carrot slices.

5. Romaine lettuce boats filled with fresh guacamole.

Favorite Supplements for Healthy Aging

No antiaging formulas reside in a bottle, but supplements can provide nutrients you're not getting from food alone. These four proven supplements are worth the investment, like a "little extra" for your life insurance policy.

Fish oils rich in omega-3 fatty acids reduce inflammation and protect the cell membrane from oxidative damage. They are one of the few supplements we highly recommend for its many age-reversing benefits.

Dose: Common fish oil capsules found in health food stores contain approximately 180 mg of DHA and 120 mg of EPA; however, 1,000-3,000 mg of DHA/EPA from fish oil is recommended. If you don't like to take fish oil, consider eating Atlantic salmon, which contains about 2.5 grams of EPA/DHA per 4 oz serving.

Vitamin D. Vitamin D is a fat soluble vitamin, meaning it gets better absorbed when consumed as a supplement with food containing fat. It affects more than 200 genes in your body. It offers a broad-spectrum of health benefits, such as improving bone metabolism and immunity, reducing cognitive decline, improving mood and well-being, and decreasing your risk of all major types of cancer.

Dose: Supplement with 5,000 IU to 8,000 IU of vitamin D3 daily with fat containing food to improve absorption. Take a 25-hydroxy vitamin D blood test after three months to assess and adjust your dosage so your optimal blood levels stay between 50–80 ng/mL year-round.

Coenzyme Q10. Coenzyme Q10 (CoQ10 for short) is a potent antioxidant and is most concentrated in the cells of your body's "workhorse" organs—like your brain and your heart. It is essential for healthy energy production within the mitochondria—the cell's energy powerhouse—where it converts the energy from fats and sugars into energy that is usable by the cells. It can improve blood sugar levels, insulin resistance, blood pressure, and improve your cholesterol markers.

Dose: Aim for 60-100mg/day.

Collagen. Collagen is the single most abundant protein in our bodies—it's the glue that holds everything together and can be found in your muscles, skin, bones, joints, and tendons. Collagen strengthens your skin and helps replace dead skin cells. As you age, you produce less collagen, which triggers wrinkles, weaker cartilage in the joints, and sagging, aging skin. Consuming optimal amounts of protein from clean sources such as wild caught fish and legumes provides the essential amino acid building blocks for collagen. But using it as a supplement can help provide the amount needed to rebuild your connective tissue and keep your skin more elastic.

Dose: Simply add 1-2 tablespoons of collagen powder into your smoothies, coffee, or green tea each day. Collagen is protein and delivers approximately 6 grams of protein per scoop. You can find collagen powder sold at most health food stores.

Daily Food Practices that Can Reverse Aging

Intermittent Fasting. There's a growing body of research showing that fasting can have beneficial effects on our general health. *We need to cue our bodies to shut down appropriately at night. Our organs need adequate rest to digest the day's meals and to heal, and they can't do this well if we're indulging in late-night cravings. An "overnight" fast between twelve and sixteen hours between dinner and breakfast helps ensure better elimination, hormone balance, and even sound circadian rhythms, which is regulating your internal body clock.*

Through rest, the body can repair tissues in the liver and pancreas and improve a number of potent disease factors. For example, modern science has confirmed fasting can help:

- Normalize your insulin sensitivity and reduce insulin resistance
- Normalize ghrelin levels, also known as "the hunger hormone"
- Promote human growth hormone (HGH) production which is produced in the pituitary gland and plays a vital role in cell regeneration, growth and maintaining healthy human tissue, including the brain and various vital organs.

- Lower triglyceride levels. Triglycerides are a fat that can be used for short term energy; however, elevated levels are associated with heart disease and metabolic health issues
- Reduce inflammation and free radical damage

Practice eating within an eight-hour window and fast for sixteen hours. For example, aim to finish your dinner between 6 and 8 p.m., and then eat your next meal between 10 a.m. and noon the following day. Do this once or twice per week for weight loss and to boost your longevity genes. *Over time, you may graduate to doing this four to five days a week and take a break on the weekends. You'll be surprised at how one small change like this can greatly improve your health in a short period of time.*

Buy Seasonal and Local Produce

Although our expansive, modern supermarkets stock produce year-round, many items travel thousands of miles to reach the shelves. To enjoy the true taste of produce, visit your local farmers' market and acquaint yourself with what's available seasonally. You'll find the produce is not only a better value, but it tastes so much better, too. This may motivate you to eat more of the colorful foods that can help you age well.

Grow Some of Your Own Food

You don't have to own a farm to grow your own herbs and a few veggies. All you need is a sunny windowsill and a few pots to start your own patch of basil, rosemary or thyme, and garlic. The benefit is that fresh herbs are packed with more flavor and age-reversing antioxidants than dried herbs. Plus, you benefit from the reward and satisfaction of growing and eating your own food.

Conclusions

Wherever you are on the continuum of aging, remember that you can optimize your healthspan through your daily food and lifestyle choices. Hopefully, some of the ideas shared here will inspire you to incorporate more healing, colorful foods, reduce some of the inflammatory foods, add a few supplements and even grow a little of your own food to help you live as long and as well, as possible!

References

Ornish D, et al. Changes in gene expression in men undergoing an intensive nutrition and lifestyle intervention. *Proc Natl Acad Sci U S A*. 2008 Jun 17;105(24): 8369– 74.

Vistoli, G., et al. "Advanced glycoxidation and lipoxidation end products (AGEs and ALEs): an overview of their mechanisms of formation." Free Radical Research 47 (August, 2013): Supplement 1:3.

Guilbaud, A., et al. "How Can Diet Affect the Accumulation of Advanced Glycation End-Products in the Human Body?" Foods 5 no. 4 (2016): pii: E84.

Kellow, N.J., et al. "Effect of diet-derived advanced glycation end products on inflammation." Nutrition Review 73 no. 11 (2015): 737-59.

Fonseca, Vivian A. "Defining and Characterizing the Progression of Type 2 Diabetes." *Diabetes Care* 32 no. 2 (2009): S151–S156.

Lau, C., et al. "Dietary glycemic index, glycemic load, fiber, simple sugars, and insulin resistance: the Inter99 study." *Diabetes Care* **28 no. 6** (2005): 1397-403.

Ding M, Satija A, Bhupathiraju SN, Hu Y, Sun Q, Han J, Lopez-Garcia E, Willett W, van Dam RM, Hu FB. Association of Coffee Consumption with Total and Cause-Specific Mortality in 3 Large Prospective Cohorts. Circulation. 2015 Dec 15;132(24):2305-15.

Gunter MJ, Murphy N, Cross AJ, Dossus L, Dartois L, et.al. Coffee Drinking and Mortality in 10 European Countries: A Multinational Cohort Study. Ann Intern Med. 2017.

Park SY, Freedman ND, Haiman CA, Le Marchand L, Wilkens LR, Setiawan VW. Association of Coffee Consumption With Total and Cause-Specific Mortality Among Nonwhite Populations. Ann Intern Med. 2017 Jul 11.

Biofactors. 2003;18(1-4):91-100. Conclusions

Genome Res. 2010 Oct;20(10):1352-60.

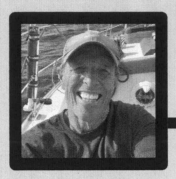

DR. THOMAS W. STORER completed undergraduate and graduate programs in kinesiology and exercise science at California State University and a PhD in exercise science at the University of Utah. He has taught and conducted research at the college and university levels for more than thirty-five years. His research has focused on androgens, resistance exercise training, and other function-promoting therapies to combat the muscle wasting and physical dysfunction common in aging, obesity, and chronic disease. Dr. Storer's interests extend to clinical applications of cardiopulmonary exercise testing and interpretation and their use in interventions for improving aerobic function and performance.

He currently serves as Director of the Exercise Physiology and Physical Performance Laboratory and as Associate Director of the Functional Assessment Core, Claude Pepper Older Americans Independent Center, at Brigham and Women's Hospital in Boston, MA. He is the author or coauthor of more than one hundred peer reviewed publications. He has served as Chief Exercise Physiologist for the National Institute on Aging-funded Testosterone Trials and other NIH- and industry-funded trials of anabolic interventions for improved physical function. He is now co-chair of the Physical Components Subcommittee for the STRIDE fall prevention study and Chair of the Physical Function Sub-study for the Football Players Health Study at Harvard. He is an avid sailor and exercise enthusiast.

CHAPTER 6

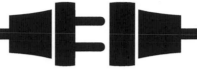

Taking Care of Muscle—The Engines that Move You

by DR. THOMAS W. STORER

Skeletal muscles are indeed the engines that move us. They also provide the ability to lift, push, pull, carry, and hold objects including our own body weight. The size, strength, power, and endurance of muscles allow us to perform activities that require these functions with ease and enjoyment or with difficulty, or in some cases, not at all. Aging brings about several changes in our muscle physiology and ability to function physically. This deterioration with age is normal but inactivity accelerates the process. In the worst cases, aging and disuse may lead to disability and loss of independence. No one wants that.

Think back 10, 20, 30, 40, or 50 years. Remember the tasks that you were able to accomplish with relative ease? Are these now more difficult? Have you stopped activities that you really enjoyed because they became too difficult, you thought they were unsafe, or you just lost interest in them? Some might answer yes, it's difficult so I just won't do that anymore; or, "It's easier to take the elevator/escalator"; or, "Well, I'll just live downstairs since going up my staircase is too difficult." And, "What if there is a fire or other emergency and I can't get down the stairs? I'm worried about whether I might fall."

Are you able to rise from the floor with ease? Can you carry groceries, suitcases, grandchildren? When on vacation, are you able to enjoy the wonderful sights that might require some walking or stair climbing? Is hiking or playing tennis or bicycling now off your interest list because you question your physical ability?

What if you could get back those abilities? It's not a matter of *if* because you *can*; it's the how-to, the motivation, and use of specific types of exercise training that are important. You <u>will be</u> successful! Resistance exercise training, even a little bit done regularly, will enhance muscle function and lead the way to improved physical function.

This chapter will first provide definitions of key terms that will be used throughout the chapter. We will then briefly explore the many benefits that come about with resistance exercise training. These are important to know because people tend to be motivated by those things that provide value and meaning to their lives. Some, if not all, of the benefits available through resistance training should resonate with you and thought of as important. We will look at what goes on with our skeletal muscles as we age, why we become less able, and review a few ideas on how every day, simple activities can slow down the loss of function. After these preliminaries, we will examine the methods, the "how tos" with which we can apply resistance exercise training, using evidence-based guidelines to improve physical function. How about a little evidence right now for how resistance training can improve muscle function and physical performance?

Dr. Maria Fiatarone and colleagues provided just 8 weeks of supervised resistance exercise training to a sample of 10 frail residents of a rehabilitation hospital for the aged in Boston, MA.[1] The male and female subjects averaged 90 years of age! These subjects performed resistance exercise training with a leg-extension exercise on 3 days each week with 3 sets of 8 repetitions, progressively increasing resistance over the 8 weeks. Nine individuals completed the study. Remarkably, these subjects averaged a 174% increase in leg strength, a 9% increase in the muscle area of the thigh, and a 48% increase in walking speed over 6 meters, about 20 feet. This is not an isolated study. Several other studies in older men and women have reported similar findings. **Table 1** provides a list of additional benefits that might be expected from regular resistance training.

Table 1. Benefits from Regular Exercise Training

• Improves muscle strength 25-100% or more	• Slows, stops, or reverses bone loss
• Activities we do every day are easier	• Improves self-confidence
• Improves muscle tone and firmness	• Improves self-efficacy
• Can increase muscle power	• Improves self-esteem

• Increases endurance	• Helps to maintain independence
• Improves posture	• Improves quality of life
• Decreases risk of falls including injurious falls	• Reduces mortality risk from all causes

We can summarize these benefits in a few words: feel better, look better, do more, live longer, stay independent.

Definitions

- **Muscle strength**: The maximal force a particular muscle can exert; the maximal resistance that can be moved one time only.
- **Muscle power**: How fast a muscle exerts force; important in activities of daily living (ADL) and recreational activities.
- **Muscle endurance**: How many times a muscle can move an object (including your body weight!) before it fatigues, or how long the muscle can hold an object, like a bag of groceries.
- **Lean body mass (LBM)**: All parts of the body other than fat; LBM includes muscle, bone, ligaments, tendons, organs, fluids, skin, and hair.
- **Skeletal muscle mass (SMM)**: A part of the LBM that provides the "engine" to move or hold with the aid of tendons, ligaments, and bone.
- **Atrophy**: Loss of LBM, especially SMM. Loss of SMM is often due to disuse, aka "disuse atrophy."
- **Hypertrophy**: In the context of this chapter, *hypertrophy* refers to muscle growth; an increase in the size of muscles.

Increased muscle size is generally associated with increased muscle strength.

- **Sarcopenia:** The age-related loss of muscle mass associated with disuse atrophy, poor protein and energy intake, loss of motor neurons, change in hormonal status, chronic diseases, and inflammation.

- **1-RM:** A measure of strength; the maximal amount of weight that can be moved one time only.

- **Set:** A group of repetitions, for example, 10.

- **Repetition:** The complete cycle of moving a resistance from its starting point to the end of the range of motion and back to the starting point.

- **Load intensity:** An indication of the level of effort required to perform a repetition or set. Load can take the form of the weight of a dumbbell or barbell, body weight, the resistance from elastic tubing, and so on.

- **Progression:** The systematic increase over time in the frequency, number of sets and repetitions, load, and number of exercises. Progression is necessary to continue improvement.

Skeletal Muscle and Aging

Muscle mass declines about 30% from twenty to eighty years of age. An example of this decline is shown in the two images in **Figure 1.** Each image is a cross-sectional slice through the thigh muscle. The central black area is the thigh bone (femur), and the gray areas are muscle. The light-colored areas are fat. The image on the left is from an individual 25 years of age; the image on the right from a person 63 years or age. Note the decreased gray areas on the right indicating loss of muscle mass. Also note the increase in the light areas on the right, which indicate increased fat mass, including that seen within the muscle itself. As you might expect, such a loss of muscle mass affects muscle strength, power, endurance, and even metabolism. This loss of muscle mass and function is known as sarcopenia, a highly prevalent condition in older individuals that can lead to functional decline and disability.

Figure 1. Cross section of thigh showing bone (central back area), muscle (gray areas), and fat (light areas).
Left panel from a person 25 years of age.
Right panel from an individual 63 years of age.

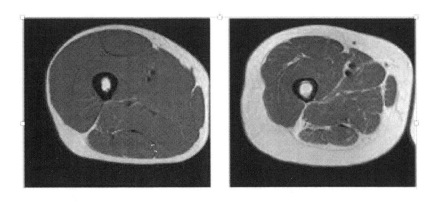

Is it possible to avoid sarcopenia, regain muscle mass, and function? Absolutely. To the ladies who may be reading this chapter, please put out of your mind any thoughts of how the exercise described here might make your muscles big and bulky. This is not going to happen. First, you don't have enough testosterone, the male hormone that helps increase muscle size and strength; most women have only about 10% of the average male value. Also, following the training guidelines below will not result in big, bulky muscles. Honest!

An individual's *muscle strength* (see "Definitions") is greatest at about 25-30 years of age. People who have been active and stay active in resistance exercise training tend to maintain that peak to about age forty then experience a very gradual decline to age sixty at which point the decline accelerates as shown in **Figure 2.** People who don't exercise regularly begin to progressively lose strength after age thirty so that by age sixty-five they have lost 25-30% of the strength they had at age thirty. By age eighty, untrained individuals will have lost almost 60% of the strength they had at age thirty whereas the person who regularly resistance trains will have lost only about 25%.

Figure 2. Changes in knee extensor strength with aging in men who have regularly strength trained versus untrained men.

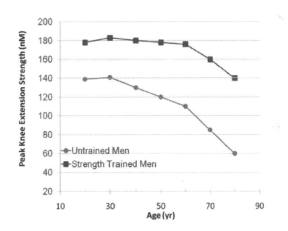

Muscle power (see "Definitions"), particularly in the legs, decreases at an even faster rate than strength. This is because the muscle fibers that are especially suited for power are lost (atrophy) faster than others. This loss has significant impact one's ability to do every day functional tasks and recreational activities because muscle power is more well associated with these activities than strength. We lose the power fibers faster as we age because we simply do not "ask" them to contract! Developing or maintaining muscle power requires them to contract rapidly against a load. Examples include climbing stairs or standing up from a chair. You can improve your lower extremity muscle power in a couple of easy ways. When rising from a seated position, try to do it quickly four, five, or more times. When climbing stairs, hold the handrail and push off the steps as fast as possible. You do not have to do this for every step, but begin with one to three steps and progress safely as you become more able.

Here's another exercise mantra applied to stairs: "Up one, down two. Take the stairs, they're good for you." When you have the option of stairs, elevator, or escalator, walk up one flight of stairs, then switch to mechanical means if you like. When descending, try to walk down (hold the handrail!) at least two floors.

With all this information about muscle loss, decline in physical function with age, and encouragement to improve muscle function, are older adults actually participating in resistance exercise training? Sadly, no. The most recent data available from the Centers for Disease Control and Prevention report that only 4.5% of adults aged sixty-five to seventy-four and 5.8% of adults over age seventy-four met the 2008 federal guidelines for resistance exercise training.

As you will see in more detail below, these guidelines suggest 2 days per week or more of resistance exercise training that includes at least one set of 10-15 repetitions with a moderate load for 8-10 exercises. You will also see that depending on how the workout sessions are constructed throughout the week, fulfilling these guidelines could take as little as eight minutes.

But the central question is, how do I perform an effective resistance exercise program? Let's answer that question.

Evidence-Based Guidelines for Resistance Exercise Training

Strong evidence from multiple, well-designed research studies over many years support the value of resistance exercise training and have guided program design. The most current evidence-based guidelines for resistance exercise training in both younger and older adults come from the *2017 American College of Sports Medicine Guidelines for Exercise Testing and Prescription* [2] and are shown in **Table 2.** The *frequency, intensity, sets, repetitions, rest,* and *number of exercises* may be considered as a reasonable starting point for most healthy people. Let's dive a little deeper into these recommendations.

Table 2. Evidence-Based Guidelines for Resistance Exercise Training in Healthy Younger and Older Adults

Age Group	Frequency	Intensity	Sets	Repetitions	Rest	Number of Exercises
Adults 18-65 yr.	≥ 2 d/wk	Volitional fatigue*	1	8-12	60 seconds	8-10
Older, healthy adults	≥ 2 d/wk	Moderate 5/10 High 7/10	≥1	10-15	60 seconds	8-10

* *Volitional fatigue* may be considered as when one cannot perform another repetition in good form or chooses not to because of fatigue.

Frequency: The recommended frequency of training is at least two days per week. But this needs some clarification. This two-day-per-week recommendation presumes that the individual will train all of the major muscle groups (**Table 3**) on each of the two days. This is the most commonly recommended program.

Table 3. Major Muscle Groups

Body Part	Muscle names
Front thigh muscles	Quadriceps
Back thigh muscles	Hamstrings
Calf muscles	Gastrocnemius and soleus
Abdomen	Rectus abdominis, obliques, transverse abdominis
Lower back muscles	Erector spinae
Chest muscles	Pectoralis major and minor
Midback muscles	Latissimus dorsi
Upper-back muscles	Trapezius and rhomboids
Shoulder muscles	Deltoids
Arms	Biceps and triceps

However, some people may prefer to split the number of muscle groups trained on a given day. (This does save time when you think in terms of the time and energy investments in single-exercise sessions.) One way to split the training is to do half of the muscle groups, four or five muscle groups, on two days, perhaps Monday and Thursday, while the other four or five muscle groups are exercised on two other days, such as Tuesday and Friday (see **Table 4A**).

Another way to split resistance training is over six days where three to four muscle groups are exercised each day (see **Table 4B**). Some individuals like the six-day split because it helps form the habit of exercising six out of seven days each week. Here are some examples of four- and six-day split routines. Note that each major muscle group receives training two days per week; there is always two days of rest between exercising the same muscle group; and exercises on each day are arranged so as not to overly fatigue a given muscle group. These are but two examples of the many ways you can arrange your weekly resistance training schedule.

Table 4A. Four-Day Split Resistance Exercise Routine

Monday	Tuesday	Wednesday	Thursday	Friday	Saturday (Rest)	Sunday (Rest)
Quadriceps	Pectorals		Quadriceps	Pectorals		
Hamstrings	Latissimus dorsi		Hamstrings	Latissimus dorsi		
Calf	Upper back		Calf	Upper back		
Abdominals	Deltoids		Abdominals	Deltoids		
Arms	Low back		Arms	Lower back		

Table 4B. Example of a Six-Day Split Routine

Monday	Tuesday	Wednesday	Thursday	Friday	Saturday	Sunday
Quadriceps	Latissimus dorsi	Pectorals	Quadriceps	Latissimus dorsi	Pectorals	
Hamstrings	Upper back	Deltoids	Hamstrings	Upper back	Deltoids	
Biceps	Abdominals	Lower back	Biceps	Abdominals	Lower back	
Triceps	Calf		Triceps	Calf		

Helpful hints:

- Provide at least two days per week of resistance exercise for each major muscle group
- Avoid training the same muscle group two days in a row. The more recovery time between workouts, the better.

- Start with the largest muscle groups scheduled and proceed to the smallest.
- Arrange training and rest days to best fit your personal schedule.
- Modify as needed.

Intensity: This is the "How hard?" part, the level of exertion recommended during the workout. For younger, healthy people, "volitional fatigue" is the guideline. This means that at the end of a set of 12 repetitions, the exerciser should not be able to do a 13th rep in good form. The 8-12 repetition guideline indicates that a person should choose a resistance that in good form and full range of motion can be done at least 8 times but not more than 12 times. For older, healthy adults, the *intensity* of an exercise is rated on a point scale from 0 to 10 with 5 indicating moderate exertion. This is the intensity with which older adults should begin. As the individual becomes regular in his or her training over several weeks and progress is made, part or all of the training could be done at a 7, which is a vigorous level of exertion. This level should be approached with caution. In most cases, the only negative effect of resistance training is getting injured. Injury will not only keep a person from training, it will also result in losing some of the previous gains. A good exercise mantra for older adults is *start low, go slow*. Good advice.

Sets and Repetitions: The recommendation for older, healthy adults is one or more sets of 10-15 reps. It is prudent to begin with a single set for each exercise and then add sets when you are ready and it is safe to do so. Remember, *"start low, go slow."* A *repetition* of an exercise represents the complete up and down, in and out, forward and backward cycle of the exercise. For example, a repetition of an arm curl for the biceps starts with the arms hanging down and holding dumbbells or other resistance equipment in the hands, raising the weight to the shoulder, pausing momentarily, then lowering the weight to the starting position, pausing briefly, and repeating for the specified number of reps. How fast you raise and lower the resistance weight is also important. Typically, the up-and-down parts should take about 2 seconds each, and the total time for the pauses is 1-2 seconds. Each rep should take 5-6 seconds, or about a minute to a minute and a half for one set of an exercise. This guideline may be useful when deciding on how many exercises one wishes to include in an exercise session. Using a 2-day per week routine, 10 exercises with the recommended 1-minute rest between exercises adds up to a 20- to 25-minute exercise session. A 4-day split would take 10-15 minutes each day, and a 6-day split would require about 8-10 minutes per session.

Rest Interval: In the last section on sets and reps, we indicated that a one-minute rest interval between sets is appropriate and often adequate for most healthy older adults. However, if you feel the need to rest longer, by all means do so! Specifying the rest interval is actually important when one progresses to two sets or more of an exercise. Too little rest will result in earlier fatigue; longer rest will not provide an appropriate challenge to using more of the muscle in the exercise.

Number of Exercises: Guidelines suggest 8-10 resistance training exercises using the frequency, sets, repetitions, and rest intervals discussed above. This represents one exercise for each of the major muscle groups as shown in **Table 4.** This is an excellent starting point for most healthy, older adults, but some people who are not in very good condition could start with fewer exercises.

Lower-extremity exercises are important for increasing mobility and balance and are directly applicable to improving functional ability, such as rising from a chair, the bed, or toilet seat; climbing stairs; and walking. Arm and shoulder exercises are useful in lifting, holding, and carrying objects. In addition, exercises for these muscle groups require less equipment and are easier to integrate into the daily routine. Examples of good leg-strengthening exercises include sitting and standing from a chair 10-15 times, or raising yourself up on your toes 10-15 times while holding onto the kitchen counter or brushing your teeth.

Training for Power: Earlier in this chapter, the recommended speed of each repetition was said to be a total of about 5-6 seconds; in a stand-up exercise, this means 2 seconds for sitting, a brief pause, and then 2 seconds to stand up, followed by another brief pause before the next repetition. This is a safe and effective speed and the advisable speed of movement particularly as you begin training. However, after 4-6 weeks of twice-weekly exercises, your muscles will have adapted to the point where you might introduce some power training. We know that power is important for improving physical function, especially lower-extremity function.[3,4,5]

Let's use the sit-to-stand exercise again as an example. You should still lower yourself slowly, taking about two seconds, to the chair seat, but instead of standing up after the pause, stand as quickly as possible to your full height, pause, and repeat. Power comes from that very rapid contraction of the muscles during the standing movement. Another example is climbing stairs. When your lead foot hits the next step, push off the step as quickly as possible. Be sure to hold the handrail for support!

Power training is best suited for lower-extremity exercise for most people because of its direct association with everyday physical function. Introduce power training gradually and only after 4-6 weeks of initial training. Limiting power training to one of the 2 days of training per week is a good way to start.

Progression and Overload: When used in the context of resistance exercise training, overload is a good thing! *Overload* means increasing the demands on the muscle during training that are greater than the muscle is used to doing. In 1951, Thomas DeLorme, a US Army surgeon, developed a method of exercise training that was called Progressive Resistance Exercise.[6] Progressive resistance training, or PRT, is a process of progressively increasing the resistance (load) during training to overcome the muscle's natural ability to adapt to the previous load. This method is used throughout the world as a basis for resistance training.

One application of the method is to increase the resistance by 5-10% for upper-body exercises and 10-20% for lower-body exercises. For example, when one is able to complete all planned repetitions (let's say 15 repetitions) for three consecutive workouts, the resistance can be increased. Another way to progress is by adding another set to the exercises. The overarching objective is to provide progressive overload so that the muscle continues to grow and *increase* function.

When do you get to stop progressing? One answer is when you have reached your training objective and wish to just maintain newfound gains of muscle growth, muscle performance, and physical function. This is a good answer so long as it is consistent with optimizing your physical function.

Warm-up: The *warm-up* before training is for the purpose of increasing blood flow and thus heat to the muscles. Warmer muscles perform better and are less prone to injury than colder muscles. A warm-up for the lower extremity could be a 5-minute walk, cycling on a stationary cycle, or performing a few repetitions of the exercise that you are about to do using light resistance. This is referred to as a *warm-up set* and the typical way that upper-body warm-ups are done. Stretching is often thought of as part of the warm-up. You can do this if you wish, but it will not contribute to increasing the temperature of the muscle. In fact, stretching is best done after the muscle is already warm! This could include between sets of an exercise.

There you have it. Evidence-based guidelines that provide a template for a resistance-exercise-training program design. But, we have other issues to deal with, right? For example, what do I need to do to get started? I understand which body parts and muscles need to be trained, but what exercises are best? Do I have to go to a gym? Can I do the exercises at home? Do I have to buy equipment? What are the safety concerns? Should I see my doctor first? These are all reasonable and practical questions that can be successfully addressed.

Getting Started

We will all have different starting points based on our exercise history and current exercise activity, general health, physical limitations, and time availability. The guidelines shown in **Table 2** are targeted toward healthy individuals. Those with chronic diseases, including heart disease, lung disease, cancer, diabetes, and others can and *should* include resistance exercise training as part of their lifestyle. Individuals with chronic disease should discuss resistance training with their primary care physician or specialist. Specialized resistance training program guidelines are available for most people with chronic diseases.

A good place to start is to ask yourself, "How much time to I have available to work out?" We discussed earlier in the chapter that we could have effective training routines by training 20-25 minutes twice a week, 10-15 minutes four times a week, or 8-10 minutes six times a week. If you must travel someplace to exercise, the two-day per week schedule might be best. But if your strength training is done at home, the 4- or 6-day per week routine could work well.

Pre-participation Health Screening: Resistance exercise training has been shown to be safe when properly administered even in those with chronic diseases such as heart disease, COPD, kidney disease, cancer, and others. However, it would be prudent to evaluate your current health status before starting a training program and to adhere to the safety guidelines presented later in this chapter. The American College of Sports Medicine has provided algorithms for pre-participation health screening. These are available at http://www.elementssystem.com/pdfs/Riebe.pdf).

Summarizing these guidelines, people without known cardiovascular, metabolic (e.g., diabetes), or kidney disease or their symptoms do not need approval from a health-care professional to engage in moderate exercise. Initially, light-to-moderate exercise is recommended, but intensity may progress to vigorous intensity as long as you are following guidelines. Those currently participating in regular exercise who DO have known cardiovascular, metabolic, or kidney disease but are asymptomatic may also participate in moderate-intensity exercise. All others should seek medical advice. In the absence of medical advice, individuals may use a self-screening tool called the PAR-Q+. This tool is available at http://eparmedx.com/?page_id=79.

Guidance: Enlisting an expert in resistance exercise training such as a trained, experienced, and certified personal trainer, exercise physiologist, or physical therapist to help set up and supervise your initial workouts is a good idea. This will help to ensure that you perform the exercises safely and with the best technique. As you progress, you can graduate to performing them on your own, even at home.

Equipment and Exercises: There is an enormous variety of exercises available for each muscle group. There is also a great variety in equipment, including your body weight, that can be used for resistance training. As you advance in your training, changing exercises for a particular muscle group is a good idea and part of intermediate and advanced training. However, it is beyond the scope of this book to present this programming variable here. Typical exercises are given in **Table 5** for body weight resistance exercise and for some of the common types of resistance training equipment. These are mainstays of resistance exercise training, have lower risk, are technically easier to perform, and can be used with more commonly available equipment. An excellent resource for instruction, including video clips, on how to safely and correctly perform these and many other resistance training exercises may be found on the Internet at https://www.exrx.net. Resistance exercises using *elastic resistance* such as TheraBand˚ or elastic tubing can be found on the Internet at http://www.band-exercises.net/index.html.

Table 5. Beginning Resistance Exercises for Major Muscle Groups Using Different Forms of Resistance

Muscle	Body Weight	Elastic Resistance	Dumbbells	Machine Resistance
• Quadriceps	• Rising from a seat ¼ or ½ squats, lunges	• Squats, rising from a seat, lunges, leg extension	• Squats, lunges, step-ups	• Leg press, leg extension
• Hamstrings	• Bridging	• Leg curls		• Seated leg curls

Muscle	Body Weight	Elastic Resistance	Dumbbells	Machine Resistance
• Gastrocnemius/ Soleus	• Heel rises	• Heel rises	• Heel rises	• Toe press
• Abdominals	• Sit-backs, crunch or partial crunch	• Seated or kneeling crunch		• Seated crunch
• Erector spinae	• Kneeling alternate arm and leg extension ("Bird Dog")	• Kneeling alternate arm and leg extension ("Bird Dog")	• 1 arm, bent over row, lying row	• Back extension, seated row
• Pectorals	• Push-ups, knee push-up, wall push-ups	• Push-ups, seated or standing chest press	• Supine or incline chest press	• Seated chest press
• Latissimus dorsi	• Assisted pull-up	• Seated rowing, pull-downs	• Lying row	• Front pull-down
• Trapezius/ Rhomboids		• Reverse fly	• 1 arm, bent over row	
• Deltoids	• Push-ups, knee push-up, wall push-ups	• Lateral rise	• Lateral rise	• Lateral rise
• Biceps		• Arm curls	• Arm curls	• Arm curls
• Triceps	• Push-ups, knee push-up, wall push-ups; bent knee partial dips	• Triceps extension	• Triceps extension	• Triceps extension

NOTE: Many of these exercises may be unfamiliar to you. Before starting. Be sure to seek guidance from a qualified expert. Refer to https://www.exrx.net and http://www.band-exercises.net/index.html for more information.

Monitoring and Record Keeping

Keeping records, which can be as simple as notations on a calendar, is a well-accepted motivational strategy. Recording what you have done is inspiring! It shows your accomplishments and helps you plan future workouts as you progress. The progress you see will also help set or readjust your training goals. Be sure to note how your resistance training has impacted your physical function and quality of life. If your journal has not revealed improvements after a few weeks of training, look more deeply into what you have done, analyze your efforts, and possibly return to this chapter and modify your training as needed. Chances are you weren't following the guidelines at some level. Often, this is just the frequency of training. Remember, you can't get better unless you show up!

Safety

Injuries seen with resistance exercise training are rare particularly when supervised by trained and experienced experts. One published study[7] showed an injury rate of 0.05 per 1000 participant hours over 2.5 years; very small indeed! Greater risk of injury has been reported when training is unsupervised, especially when done in the home by inexperienced individuals. Safety can be enhanced by following these guidelines:

Use strict lifting technique. There is a right way and many wrong ways to perform an exercise. Learn and practice correct form and use it unfailingly.

Monitor breathing. One of the most important safety concerns with resistance exercise is how one breathes during each repetition. The general guideline is simple: DON'T HOLD YOUR BREATH. Holding your breath while lifting creates something called the Valsalva maneuver, which results in high pressure in the chest that increases blood pressure and reduces blood flow to the heart. Simply breathing normally during the exercise or exhaling gently when lifting and inhaling when lowering weights are good strategies.

Perform exercises through the full range of motion (ROM): A goal of resistance exercise training is to increase strength, power, or endurance over the complete distance the joint can move—the ROM. For example, when doing an arm curl with dumbbells, the weight should begin with the arm and elbow fully extended, followed by lifting the weight as far as the joint will allow, typically to the shoulder, then returning to the starting point. There are some exceptions: The squat and leg press exercises should not allow greater than 90 degrees of knee flexion for most people, especially older adults.

Monitor adverse signs and symptoms: Be constantly aware of the onset of dizziness, excessive shortness of breath, chest pain or pressure, heart rhythm irregularities, joint and muscle pain. For the latter, soreness, so long as it goes away in twenty-four to forty-eight hours, is okay. Undeniable pain is not. If any of these signs or symptoms occur during training, please rest, and consider whether resuming is safe. Best to stop and be safe so as to train another day.

A Simple 2 x 6 Plan

Ours is a complex world with many competing demands on our time and energy. In addition to resistance training, you should also include regular aerobic-type exercise (walking, jogging, cycling, rowing, to name a few) in your weekly schedule. National guidelines suggest 150 minutes per week of this activity spread out over most days. A typical way to achieve this is 30 minutes 5 days per week. Many people start off slowly and work up to 150 minutes per week as a target. However, this should be considered the minimum; 200 or even 300 minutes per week will bring better benefits.

How can we save time and still reap the many benefits of resistance exercise training? One way is the 2 x 6 plan recommended by Dr. Wayne Westcott, a world authority on practical approaches to resistance training. This method suggests 2 days per week of one set for six major muscle group exercises. This workout would take 24 to 30 minutes per *week* (12-15 minutes on each of 2 days). Pretty doable! This plan works because smaller muscle groups— like the biceps, triceps, deltoids, and calves—are used to assist the large muscle groups (latissimus dorsi, pectorals, and quadriceps, respectively) used in the large muscle group exercises.

A weekly 2 x 6 plan would look something like this: On each of two days, do one set of 10-15 repetitions at a moderate effort (5 on a 0-10 scale) for the following six muscle groups: quadriceps, hamstrings, pectorals, latissimus dorsi, abdominals, and lower back. (See **Table 5** for exercise options). Progress by adding 1-2 sets or increasing resistance or both. If time becomes more available, add a day for a 3 x 6 plan and go for it!

Nutritional Support

This section suggests ways that nutrition might be adjusted to optimize muscle growth, strength, and function to combat the age-associated loss of these important characteristics that lead to *sarcopenia,* the age-related loss of muscle mass. Specifically, protein, energy, and the supplement *creatine monohydrate* will be reviewed in the context of aging and in support of resistance exercise training.

The *recommended daily allowance* (RDA) now correctly known as the Dietary Reference Intake (DRI) for protein, was set by the

Institute of Medicine at 0.8 grams per kilogram body weight per day or about 0.36 grams per pound body weight per day.[8] This DRI has been applied to adults 19–>70 years of age, male and female. Some research has shown that muscles in older individuals may experience reduced responsiveness to dietary protein in terms of using protein for building muscle. This has been called "anabolic resistance"[9] and is now under intense study. It appears that older adults who consume protein at or below the current DRI experience loss of lean body mass. However, eating more than the RDA has shown inconsistent effects on muscle and physical function.

Nevertheless, an international expert study group was recently tasked with reviewing dietary protein needs with aging—the PROT-AGE study group—to provide evidence-based recommendations for optimal dietary protein intake in older people[10]. Briefly summarizing, this group recommended that older adults (over age sixty-five) should consume 1.0 to 1.2 grams of protein per kilogram body weight, or 0.36 to 0.54 grams per pound. Protein quality should also be considered. "Fast proteins" (proteins that have faster digestion and uptake) such as whey protein are preferred over "slow proteins" such as casein and other protein sources such as soy. Older adults with chronic disease or malnutrition may need more protein in their diet. An exception is people with severe kidney disease who are not on dialysis; they should limit their protein intake.

Timing of protein intake may be important in augmenting the effects of resistance training. One study gave older men (average age was 74) a liquid supplement containing 10 grams protein, 7 grams carbohydrate, and 3 grams fat *immediately after* or *two hours after* exercise training. The men who completed 12 weeks of three-times per week resistance training and took the supplement immediately after training showed significant increases in muscle size. The men who consumed the supplement *two hours after* training showed no change in muscle size.[11] More recent data, however suggest that consuming protein and energy (carbohydrates) soon before or soon after resistance training optimizes its benefit.

While there is no consensus on the optimal protein dose, it appears that doses up to 40 grams after exercise have been effective in older individuals. Believe it or not, chocolate milk has been recommended as a good post-workout supplement! But be careful. One cup of chocolate milk can contain 30 grams (2 ½ tablespoons, 120 calories) of simple sugar and 8 grams of saturated fat (72 calories). The simple sugars are the best carbohydrates for post- workout muscle repair and building but should be limited to less than 10 % of total calories consumed per day. Saturated fat should also be limited to less than 10 % of total calories. So be aware of the need to adjust other parts of your diet.

Exercise of any type, including resistance exercise, expends energy. Energy is also required to facilitate *repair* of the microscopic muscle tears[1] that result from exercise. Energy is also required to fuel the processes that build muscle with amino acids from protein as the building blocks. Think of it this way: Your backyard brick wall (muscle) sustained some damage. You hire a brick mason and buy bricks for the repair. The mason provides the energy for the repair, and the bricks are the amino acids. You also decide to reinforce that wall so that it is bigger and stronger. The mason expends more

---

1   Don't be alarmed by the reference to muscle tears. Resistance exercise training causes slight muscle damage during the training, but this is not a bad thing unless it is wildly excessive, and in fact, muscle damage and repair is *necessary* for muscle growth. Following the guidelines provided in this chapter is not likely to result in excessive muscle damage.

energy to do this, and more bricks (amino acids) are required. To be complete, you insist that the mason arrive immediately with the bricks to start work. As with the repair and fortification of the brick wall, regular resistance exercise training brings about needs for increased energy and protein intake. In summary, 10-40 grams of protein along with simple sugars consumed soon before or soon after exercise can enhance the muscle building effects of resistance training. Aiming for a total daily protein intake of about 0.45 to 0.54 grams per pound has been recommended for older adults[10].

Creatine is produced naturally in the body from three amino acids. Biochemically, creatine acts to rapidly replenish the energy used by muscles during short-term, intense contractions. This replenishment allows more energy for continued muscle contractions, which leads to more effective training and the associated gains in muscle size and strength. This biochemical action is one of the theoretical bases for creatine's potential effectiveness. Creatine is plentiful in dietary sources such as seafood and red meat. Therefore, creatine supplementation may have a less pronounced effect on muscle in people who regularly consume red meat and seafood. Creatine is also available as a dietary supplement in the form of creatine monohydrate that has been shown to increase muscle size, strength, and function in older adults. While most supplements that promise muscle growth and improved performance are ineffective, creatine monohydrate is an exception. Hundreds if not thousands of studies have evaluated the potential value of creatine supplementation on exercise training adaptations and safety[12,13]. A preponderance of scientific evidence has shown creatine monohydrate to be an effective supplement for augmenting resistance training to increase muscle size and strength[12]. Creatine has also been shown to be safe when used as directed[14]. Like most out-of-the-ordinary dietary and supplement information, it is prudent to check with a registered dietitian— preferably one with an interest in exercise training—or a physician before use.

Resistance training is a potent strategy for improving muscle structure and function. Good evidence [10,13,15,16] suggests that nutritional support in the form of adequate daily protein intake, protein-carbohydrate supplement before or after resistance training, as well as proper use of creatine monohydrate can increase the benefits from resistance training in older individuals. However, the key to improving muscle size, strength, and function is resistance exercise training. Without this, protein, energy, and creatine supplementation have little benefit.

Final Words

Aging brings about many changes including loss of muscle mass and physical function. This is a normal process and it happens to everyone. However, allowing yourself to become inactive accelerates these changes especially after age sixty. The good news is that you can slow down the deterioration and improve muscle mass and function, quality of life, longevity, and gain the benefits shown in **Table 1** *at any time of life*. As you read earlier in this chapter, even frail people in their nineties experienced significant improvements in muscle strength (174 %!) and physical function with only eight weeks of three times per week resistance training. If you are active now, please continue and progress with your training as described on page 103. If you are new to resistance training, PLEASE begin! Follow the guidelines in this chapter. Perhaps even start simply with the 2 x 6 program. What will this take? A little bit of time and a lot of regularity. Can you devote 12-15 minutes to resistance training two times a week? Of course you can! You will love the results. Aging is inevitable. Quality aging is a choice. What's yours?

References

1. **Fiatarone MA, Marks EC, Ryan ND, Meredith CN, Lipsitz LA, Evans WJ.** High-intensity strength training in nonagenarians. Effects on skeletal muscle. *JAMA* 1990;263(22):3029–3034.

2. **American College of Sports Medicine, Riebe D, Ehrman JK, Liguori G, Magal M, eds.** *ACSM's guidelines for exercise testing and prescription.* Tenth edition. Philadelphia: Wolters Kluwer; 2018.

3. **Pereira A, Izquierdo M, Silva AJ, Costa AM, Bastos E, González-Badillo JJ, Marques MC.** Effects of high-speed power training on functional capacity and muscle performance in older women. *Exp. Gerontol.* 2012;47(3):250–255.

4. **Ramírez-Campillo R, Castillo A, de la Fuente CI, Campos-Jara C, Andrade DC, Álvarez C, Martínez C, Castro-Sepúlveda M, Pereira A, Marques MC, Izquierdo M.** High-speed resistance training is more effective than low-speed resistance training to increase functional capacity and muscle performance in older women. *Exp. Gerontol.* 2014;58:51–57.

5. **Reid KF, Fielding RA.** Skeletal Muscle Power: A Critical Determinant of Physical Functioning in Older Adults. *Exerc. Sport Sci. Rev.* 2012;40(1):4–12.

6. **Progressive Resistance Exercise: Technic and Medical Application.** *J. Am. Med. Assoc.* 1951;146(6):606.

7. **Morrey MA, Hensrud DD.** Risk of medical events in a supervised health and fitness facility. *Med. Sci. Sports Exerc.* 1999;31(9):1233–1236.

8. **Otten JJ, Hellwig JP, Meyers LD, eds.** *DRI, dietary reference intakes:*

the essential guide to nutrient requirements. Washington, D.C: National Academies Press; 2006.

9. **Rennie MJ.** Anabolic resistance: the effects of aging, sexual dimorphism, and immobilization on human muscle protein turnover. *Appl. Physiol. Nutr. Metab. Physiol. Appl. Nutr. Metab.* 2009;34(3):377–381.

10. **Bauer J, Biolo G, Cederholm T, Cesari M, Cruz-Jentoft AJ, Morley JE, Phillips S, Sieber C, Stehle P, Teta D, Visvanathan R, Volpi E, Boirie Y.** Evidence-based recommendations for optimal dietary protein intake in older people: a position paper from the PROT-AGE Study Group. *J. Am. Med. Dir. Assoc.* 2013;14(8):542–559.

11. **Esmarck B, Andersen JL, Olsen S, Richter EA, Mizuno M, Kjaer M.** Timing of postexercise protein intake is important for muscle hypertrophy with resistance training in elderly humans. *J. Physiol.* 2001;535(1):301–311.

12. **Forbes SC, Little JP, Candow DG.** Exercise and nutritional interventions for improving aging muscle health. *Endocrine* 2012;42(1):29–38.

13. **Kreider RB, Kalman DS, Antonio J, Ziegenfuss TN, Wildman R, Collins R, Candow DG, Kleiner SM, Almada AL, Lopez HL.** International Society of Sports Nutrition position stand: safety and efficacy of creatine supplementation in exercise, sport, and medicine. *J. Int. Soc. Sports Nutr.* 2017;14(1). doi:10.1186/s12970-017-0173-z.

14. **Shao A, Hathcock JN.** Risk assessment for creatine monohydrate. *Regul. Toxicol. Pharmacol. RTP* 2006;45(3):242–251.

15. **Jäger R, Kerksick CM, Campbell BI, Cribb PJ, Wells SD, Skwiat TM, Purpura M, Ziegenfuss TN, Ferrando AA, Arent SM, Smith-Ryan AE, Stout JR, Arciero PJ, Ormsbee MJ, Taylor LW, Wilborn CD, Kalman DS, Kreider RB, Willoughby DS, Hoffman JR, Krzykowski JL, Antonio J.** International Society of Sports Nutrition Position Stand: protein and exercise. *J. Int. Soc. Sports Nutr.* 2017;14(1). doi:10.1186/s12970-017-0177-8.

16. **Kerksick CM, Arent S, Schoenfeld BJ, Stout JR, Campbell B, Wilborn**

CD, Taylor L, Kalman D, Smith-Ryan AE, Kreider RB, Willoughby D, Arciero PJ, VanDusseldorp TA, Ormsbee MJ, Wildman R, Greenwood M, Ziegenfuss TN, Aragon AA, Antonio J. International society of sports nutrition position stand: nutrient timing. *J. Int. Soc. Sports Nutr.* 2017;14(1). doi:10.1186/s12970-017-0189-4.

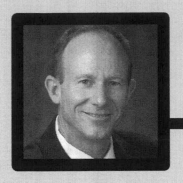

DR. WILLIAM STETSON, MD is an orthopedic surgeon in Burbank, California and has over twenty years of experience treating the orthopedic injuries of young and old alike. A former NCAA All-American volleyball player at the University of Southern California and now a fellowship-trained orthopedic surgeon specializing in sports medicine, Dr. Stetson has a unique perspective in treating those patients who want to keep moving forward and active in their lives no matter what age they are. He is an associate clinical professor of orthopedic surgery at the University of Southern California Keck School of Medicine and is also the team physician for the United States Olympic and national volleyball teams.

CHAPTER 7

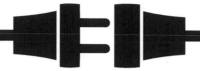

New Medical Advances for Aging Joints

By WILLIAM B. STETSON, MD

When Sharkie Zartman asked me to write this chapter, I was excited on many fronts. First and foremost was my love and respect for Sharkie and her husband, Pat. You see, Pat and Sharkie were my volleyball coaches in high school, and they taught me almost everything I know about the sport I loved and played collegiately and professionally for over twenty years. I learned from them the lessons of hard work, intensity, and perseverance that not only helped me on the volleyball court but also in the classroom as I studied to became a doctor and orthopedic surgeon. I wanted to be an orthopedic surgeon since I was twelve years old, and I am now living my dream of being a sports medicine doctor and surgeon. Having been an athlete and also a patient (I have had over ten knee surgeries and one Achilles tendon surgery), I have been on both sides of the scalpel, and so I know what it feels like to want to keep moving, playing my sports, and staying active. I hope to share in this chapter not only some of my medical knowledge but also my experience as an athlete to guide you through the maze of new possibilities for the treatment of joint problems.

With empowered aging and new advances in medical science comes some great opportunities to live longer and happier than any generation before us. In this chapter, I would like to discuss how many new medical advances for our aging joints are leading the way to keeping us more active than ever before. From dieting changes to joint supplements to better ways to exercise to new biologics and injections of our own blood (platelet rich plasma) or our own bone marrow (stem cells), these new and innovative ways to treat arthritis have the opportunity to revolutionize the treatment, and in some instances, reverse the natural aging process that occurs in all our joints.

The Basics

Before we start talking about all the new and innovative ways to treat our naturally deteriorating joints, we need to have a basic understanding of our joints and the muscles and ligaments that support them. Our joints are made up of *articular cartilage*, the smooth, glistening surfaces that glide along each other with the help of a lubricant produced by the lining of the joint, called *synovial fluid*. Think of the covering of a hard-boiled egg: The eggshell is your articular cartilage, nice and smooth, no chips, no cracks, no flaking off of the smooth shell. Unfortunately, our articular cartilage does not stay like this forever. As we age, the articular cartilage, just like the eggshell, can start to crack and flake off, causing mechanical symptoms in our knee such as painful catching and locking with swelling. This process can be accelerated with injuries to the cartilage, which can occur with a fall or a sports injury.

There are many new, innovative techniques to treat these problems, ranging from what are called *nutraceuticals* (think of them as vitamins for your joints) to different types of injections that we will also discuss to, yes, even minimally invasive surgical procedures to treat these cartilage problems. All very exciting, but wait, we can't get ahead of ourselves, we have to know the basics before we discuss what is really possible or what really is just snake oil!

We will talk a bit more about articular cartilage later in this chapter. Let's first discuss the other components of a human joint as that will give us a better understanding of what is possible.

The knee is a good example of a joint that commonly deteriorates with time and is one of the most common conditions that patients complain about and come to my office to be treated for. The knee is a hinged joint; it bends and straightens easily, but it doesn't rotate or twist very well. It has two opposing, glistening surfaces of articular cartilage—the upper part is the end of the thigh bone (*femur*) and the lower part is the top part of the shin bone (*tibia*). Sandwiched in between these two bones is the *meniscus*; there are two of them, one in the inside (*medial meniscus*) and one on the outside (*lateral meniscus*).

People often call this the *cartilage*; well, they are somewhat correct, but the knee and body have many different types of cartilage. This meniscus—which is sandwiched between the tibia (shin bone) and femur (thigh bone)—is called the *meniscal cartilage*. Don't confuse

Anterior view of the right knee

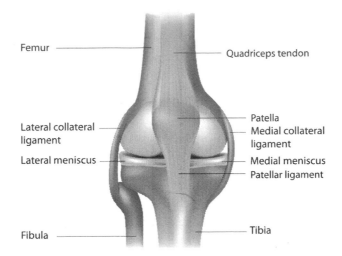

Femur — Quadriceps tendon

Lateral collateral ligament

Lateral meniscus

Patella
Medial collateral ligament
Medial meniscus
Patellar ligament

Fibula — Tibia

this with the smooth ends of the bone called the *articular cartilage;* this is a very important distinction when it comes to treatment options. So just don't assume your knee pain is due to arthritis or "cartilage damage." Have an evaluation by a health professional before you start spending your hard-earned money on treatments that have absolutely no value for your joint problems!

The knee joint, shoulder joint, hip joint, and all other joints of our body are surrounded by muscles, ligaments, and tendons that provide movement, strength, and stability for our joints. Although technically most of these are not inside our joints, they are important for overall joint health, and we will discuss why in a few minutes.

Finally, it is important to understand that all of our joints are surrounded by a structure called a *capsule.* The knee joint is the best example to use. This capsule contains the knee joint structures and the ends of the two bones that come together, which have articular cartilage at the ends of both with the menisci in between. The lining of the knee joint, like all other joints in our body, produces a liquid called synovial fluid (as previously mentioned), which lubricates this joint and allows the smooth surfaces of the articular cartilage to rub against each other with little or no friction.

What Is Arthritis?

Because most of the medical advances that we will be discussing very soon have to do with preventing, stopping, or even reversing arthritis, we need to know next exactly what *arthritis* is. Quite simply, it means inflammation of a joint. There are many different types of arthritis, however, including rheumatoid arthritis, septic arthritis, posttraumatic arthritis, and osteoarthritis. For this discussion, we are going to limit our conversation to osteoarthritis although many of the things we will discuss are applicable to these other types of arthritis also.

So what is osteoarthritis besides just inflammation of a joint? *Osteoarthritis* is what happens when our nice, smooth articular cartilages start to get worn down because, guess what, nothing lasts forever! Remember our example of the eggshell and the hard-boiled egg? That eggshell is our articular cartilage, and once it starts to crack, chip, or flake off, our bodies don't make new cartilage—bummer! So one of the first things we will talk about is how to maintain healthy joints and preserve what we already have.

Diet, Exercise, Strength, and Flexibility

Many of the medical advances we will discuss involving new "orthobiologics" have the possibility to enhance or heal joint problems caused by osteoarthritis. However, although for some this may be "the magic bullet" that they have waited so long for to cure that chronic hip or knee pain, for many others it will not work unless some basic rules of good health are followed.

First and foremost, diet, eating habits, and maintaining your weight are key! Every extra pound we carry around our belly translates to seven extra pounds of pressure to our knee joint. If we carry an extra 50 pounds of weight, that is an extra 350 pounds of pressure put on our poor knees! Extra pressure on our knees means that they will deteriorate faster; and remember, the body can't replace that articular cartilage once it is gone. Simple weight loss is the first step to maintaining healthy joints.

But what if you can't lose weight because it hurts when you exercise? I hear this every day from my patients, and it is a reasonable argument but one that is not insurmountable. Often times my patients will come to me with this complaint: They want to get in shape and lose weight, but every time they exercise, it hurts so much that they stop exercising. But guess what? They keep eating the same way! If you are truly serious about "empowered aging" and having those joints of yours survive into your eighties or nineties or even beyond, then watch what you eat and maintain a healthy diet and weight!

Hundreds of books have been written about this topic, and we have many other things to cover in this chapter. I will tell you that there is a lot that we know and don't know about the food we eat and its effect in our bodies, and in particular, on our joints. An "anti-inflammatory diet" is something to consider and is well beyond the scope of this chapter. A consult with a registered dietician is a good way to start; you may be surprised at what you learn!

Beyond our diets, there are other simple ways to maintain healthy joints before turning to more complex medical treatments, such as pills, injections, and even surgery. Regular aerobic exercise is good for our joints, along with maintaining strength and flexibility; these types of exercises will also help us keep active. Keeping the muscles that support our bodies strong is key.

Vitamins and Nutraceuticals

Okay, we covered the basics so far—diet, good nutrition, watching our weight, a simple aerobic exercise program combined with strength and flexibility—what else is out there to help us keep moving pain-free? Let's start with vitamins and other supplements called *nutraceuticals*. Many of us dismiss vitamins as not necessary if we eat a good, balanced diet—not true! Vitamin supplements such as calcium, vitamins D and B, and others are a great, simple way to keep our bones and joints strong. How do you know if you should be taking these vitamin supplements, and if so, which ones? The first step is to have an evaluation with a health-care professional. I always tell my patients they need to see their primary care physician, and if they don't have one, get one! A good primary care physician—either a family medicine doctor or an internist—is the best place to start. Along with a good physical exam, monitoring your blood pressure and other vital signs, they can do some simple blood tests to see if you are deficient in certain vitamins and also to make sure other important hormones and enzyme levels, such as your thyroid and estrogen and progesterone levels for women, testosterone levels for men, are not deficient.

Other vitamin supplements such as omega-3 fatty acids and flaxseed oil may not only be good for your joints but also for your heart by helping to keep your cholesterol down. I would urge everyone to consider adding these supplements to their vitamin regimen.

Besides vitamins, there are supplements called "nutraceuticals," which is just a fancy word for pills, liquids, or powders that may have some value, but we are not just sure what they are! One has to be careful because the claims by many of these manufacturers are not backed up by good science or research studies. They are also not controlled by the Federal Drug Administration (FDA) like prescription drugs and medicines are, so their *efficacy,* or effectiveness, may not be what they claim to be.

The one that I recommend first and foremost to my patients with joint problems, and particularly those with early or even late osteoarthritis, is glucosamine and chondroitin sulfate. These two simple substances are the building blocks of our articular cartilage, which as we discussed before, deteriorates with time either through the wear and tear of the years or through injuries. Taking this nutraceutical is supposed to "rebuild" cartilage. Well, the jury is still out on that one as many of the research studies claiming that they do rebuild cartilage were sponsored by the same manufacturers making this supplement. We still don't know if the glucosamine and chondroitin sulfates help rebuild cartilage; they may just help us keep our own joints in the status quo, or may even have a mild, safe, anti-inflammatory effect in our joints, which that in itself may help many people. I tell my patients that they are safe, may help with their knee, hip, or ankle osteoarthritis, and to try them for six months to see if they notice a difference. I would say over half my patients say they help, and with no known side effects, I say give them a try! I would add that not all of them are as pure or as well made as others, so make sure you get them from a reputable manufacturer.

There is another nutraceutical called methylsfulfonylmethane (MSM) that has shown some promise in early animal research for decreasing joint degeneration. It is an organic compound containing sulfur that may decrease the pain and swelling of knee osteoarthritis and may also help with exercise recovery. It is often combined with glucosamine and chondroitin sulfate and other joint supplements or can be found by itself. The optimal dose has not been set and varies from 500 mg three times per day to 3 grams twice per day. Again, the quality and active ingredients in these supplements may vary widely from one manufacturer to another. A MSM supplement may be worth trying for 3 months to see if you get any pain relief for those aching knees of yours. Other nutraceuticals, have not really been proven to make any differences in the health of our joints, so I would not waste my money on them.

Hyaluronic Acid Injections

Just like glucosamine and chondroitin sulfate, *hyaluronic acid* is also one of the building blocks of our articular cartilage forming what is called the *groundwork,* or *matrix,* which holds the cartilage cells in place. Glucosamine and chondroitin sulfate combined with, or attached to, a hyaluronic acid molecule forms a matrix that with collagen and cartilage cells (called *chondrocytes*) help form healthy articular cartilage. The problem we know—nothing lasts forever—and this is true for the hyaluronic acid in our joints. As we get older, less is produced, and therefore the cartilage transitions from being soft and smooth to hard and brittle. If we can "plump up" the articular cartilage and keep it from becoming brittle, possibly osteoarthritis can be prevented or just held at bay!

This is where hyaluronic acid injections can come into play and help. You might ask, why not just take a pill or supplement of hyaluronic acid instead of a shot? I hate shots! Well, if you take it by mouth, the acids in your stomach eat it up and make it useless, so it never really gets to your joints to help, so injections are the only way; sorry. But here is the good news. They can really, really help with mild, moderate, or even severe osteoarthritis, giving relief of pain for three to six months and sometimes even up to a year or longer! The science behind these injections is still somewhat vague, but please believe me, they can really work and restore your knee joint to a healthy, pain-free level of activity for an extended period of time.

Currently, these injections are only FDA approved for the knee, but doctors are allowed to use them for other joints. This practice is considered "off-label," meaning it is up to your doctor to determine if he or she thinks it will help. The problem is that insurance companies will typically pay for them if given in the knee but won't pay for them for other joints. The cost of these can be a bit pricey, ranging from $500- $1500 per injection depending on where you live and who is doing them. There are different manufacturers, and I am not about to recommend a certain brand, but I would recommend discussing this with your doctor before having them. Most are administered in a series of three, one per week for three weeks. There are a few manufacturers who are now combining all of the hyaluronic acid into a single injection—sounds great, only one shot—but I have to say we have not had much luck with these all-in-one injections, so I would stick to the once per week for three weeks.

In my clinical orthopedic surgery practice, I have been using these for over fifteen years, and it can be a real game changer for some patients, giving them long-lasting relief. It seems to be a much healthier option than cortisone (we'll get to that in a minute!), but this series often does need to be repeated every six to twelve months depending on how patients do. There is also very little downside besides a simple needle stick into the capsule of the knee, and if done with some local anesthetic like lidocaine (just like you get at the dentist), it is relatively painless. Most of these types of injections are administered by orthopedic surgeons, but other medical doctors and health-care professionals, such as physician assistants or nurse practitioners, can also safely administer them.

Steroids

"No way," you say, "not in my body!" I hear this all the time from patients and also allied health professionals as they associate steroid use with big muscles and bad side effects like growing hair in places you don't want it. Well, not always true as steroids can be very useful *if used properly*.

Let's talk real briefly about the different types of steroids—also called *corticosteroids*. Most people don't realize that our bodies produce steroids that are necessary for many different bodily functions that we take for granted. These so-called *endogenous* (made by our own bodies) *steroids*, or hormones, are important to us as they regulate everything from sexual reproduction to hair growth! So what about the *exogenous steroids* that we get them from outside our bodies via pills, creams, or even shots.

One type of exogenous steroids is *anabolic steroids,* which are used and abused by athletes to gain a competitive edge. These types of steroids can build muscle, increase strength, make you run faster and jump higher, but they have significant side effects. These types of steroids are rarely used by doctors in normal circumstances because of these horrendous side effects, which include increasing the cholesterol that causes *atherosclerosis* (hardening of the arteries), heart disease, and early death.

There are other types of steroids that, *if used properly*, can also be game changers for some people with osteoarthritis or even joint swelling of a knee joint (so-called *synovitis*, or, more simply, water on the knee) without osteoarthritis. Steroids are *fat soluble*, meaning that they can go into our bodies' cells (they can penetrate through the cell membrane and alter the nucleus of the cell) and turn on or off the mechanisms or substances that produce pain in our joints. If used properly or for the right problems, a simple, one-time injection of cortisone—for example, into the knee or hip joint— can give months and months of relief of pain, swelling, and stiffness.

The downside: These injections may not help or last as long as you would like them to. Multiple injections into one joint or location may also weaken the surrounding structures, so be careful of having too many in one spot, but they can be useful and helpful. If you do decide to have these injections, I always recommend they be accompanied by a sensible, well-structured physical therapy program under the direction of a licensed physical therapist, and eventually graduating to a continuing home exercise and strength program. Often times, a simple injection of cortisone into the knee, hip, or ankle joint will allow a patient to start a low-impact exercise program pain-free or with the pain markedly reduced. So be open to this option, but I always recommend that these types of injections be given or are under the directive of an orthopedic surgeon or another type of medical doctor well versed in the care of musculoskeletal problems.

Biologics

So far, we have covered many of the "mainstream" types of treatment for osteoarthritis, including simple exercises, strength and flexibility, nutraceutical supplements such as glucosamine and chondroitin sulfate, MSM, and even different types of injections such as hyaluronic acid and cortisone. What if none of these work or don't give you the type of pain relief you want or need to lead the active lifestyle that you want to have? What are the options? Surgery? Well, I am an orthopedic surgeon and have been doing surgery on people's shoulders, knees, hips, and ankles for over twenty years, and if done on the right patients for the right problems, surgery can be a game changer. It has a role (and we'll talk more about that later), but there are other new options to consider before surgery. These new types of treatment are of a new class called "biologics," and they have the opportunity to revolutionize the way we treat osteoarthritis and other musculoskeletal disorders.

These biologic therapies, such as platelet-rich plasma (PRP), stem cells, human amniotic membranes, and cytokines have tremendous potential for treating osteoarthritis by participating in the repair and possible regeneration of articular cartilage. These regenerative options aim to promote the body's own in vivo healing processes. However, a better understanding of the fundamental mechanisms by which all these work will help guide what roles they may play in treating or even healing osteoarthritis.

Platelet-Rich Plasma (PRP)

Most of you have heard about PRP, but you may or may not know too much about it. It starts with a health professional taking a large test tube of your own blood and placing it into a centrifuge, then spinning it around, which separates your blood into different layers. One of these layers is made up of platelets. Most of us think platelets help us only to stop bleeding; well, they do more than that or have the potential to do a lot more. Think of these *platelets* as granule-filled packets that contain multiple different types of little *cytokines,* or growth factors. These growth factors have the ability to possibly heal damaged tissue including muscles, tendons, or articular cartilage. They may have the ability to stimulate or attract new cells to help build new cartilage, or they may function as strong anti-inflammatory agents reducing or eliminating the pain and stiffness of osteoarthritis.

The problem is we need to get a better understanding of the fundamental mechanisms by which PRP exerts its effect on articular cartilage and other tissues. We are just not there yet; more research needs to be done. In the meantime, there is some evidence that PRP may help reduce the pain and stiffness from osteoarthritis; we are just not sure of the mechanism, that is, how it does this. The PRP formulations may also vary: Some are rich in white blood cells (so-called *leukocyte rich*), or some have very little numbers of white blood cells (so-called *leukocyte poor*). For the treatment of your joint pain that is caused by moderate to severe osteoarthritis, PRP, which is leukocyte poor, appears to be the best option to try. There has been some evidence from these reports in the medical literature of significant, positive results from these PRP injections for the treatment of osteoarthritis.[1]

These injections are still considered experimental, and because of that, they are not covered by your health insurance. They can be quite expensive and vary widely in price depending on where you live; for example, they cost $200 per injection in Alabama versus an average of over $1000 per injection in metropolitan areas such as New York or Los Angeles. The number of injections and how much time between injections are purely guesswork at this point in time. For now, if other treatments have failed, a single leukocyte poor PRP injection is a reasonable option to try for a significantly arthritic joint, and it may help a lot and allow you to stave off surgery, including a joint replacement.

Stem Cells

This is by far the most exciting new frontier in medicine and has the potential to be a game changer for many different maladies, including the treatment of osteoarthritis. The use of stem cells is one of the new, emerging *regenerative therapy* options for the loss of articular cartilage that occurs with osteoarthritis. The stem cells may directly participate in the repair response of damaged tissue or cartilage by being integrated into the healing tissue; they may simply have a stimulating effect by attracting the body's own cells to the site to help heal damaged tissue; or they may have an *immunomodulation effect* by stimulating the body's immune response to heal the damage. Gaining a better understanding of the fundamental mechanisms by which stem cells exert a positive effect on the body will help guide their appropriate use. The poor, intrinsic healing potential of articular cartilage makes stem cells an exciting possible treatment option for osteoarthritis. This cutting-edge technique is now being used more than ever as these treatments are touted as offering the latest and greatest way to treat an array of musculoskeletal problems, including osteoarthritis. But where do the stem cells come from, and do they really do all that they are supposed to do?

Well, good questions; let's look at the facts. *Stem cells* are "unspecialized" cells in our body that have the ability to develop into a wide variety of "specialized" cells for specific tissues or organs of the body. They can replicate or reproduce many times over, and they can even regenerate to aid in the replacement of damaged cells. The renewal properties of stem cells can be utilized to generate cells for tissue repair and the treatment of disease.

Stem cells come from different parts of the body and are also derived from different sources. *Embryonic stem cells* come from embryos in early development and have the ability to develop into any type of cell in the initial stages of development. *Fetal stem cells* come from a fetus as the maturing embryo develops and are found in fetal tissues, bone marrow, and blood. They have the potential to develop into almost any type of cell. *Umbilical cord blood stem cells* are derived from umbilical cord blood, and they can also develop into specialized cells. *Placental stem cells* are found within the placenta and can also develop into specialized stem cells. Finally, *adult stem cells* are present in mature tissues in infants, children, and adults. They are specific to a particular tissue or organ and produce the cells within that particular tissue or organ. There are many different subgroups of stem cells, and without getting too technical, they have the ability to differentiate or turn into almost anything! But what turns them on and off, or what makes them turn into a specific type of cell? Good questions, and that is where much of good medical research is being done.

Adult stem cells can be found in our bone marrow, and also, of all places, in our fat; who knew?! By harvesting them from our bone marrow or our fat, spinning them down similarly to what is done with PRP (platelet rich plasma), the stem cells are separated and concentrated and then injected, and viola, new cartilage, right? Wrong! It is just not that simple; we are still not sure what the mechanism is by which these stem cells differentiate or turn into new cartilage cells or other types of cells. But if you believe all of the advertising and promotion done over the Internet, social media, or the press, stem cells are the cure for everything! This is all for the price of anywhere from $5,000 to $10,000 per injection! We are just not there yet as we need more research to understand the best way to use this potentially effective treatment. In the meantime, I recommend to my patients that they first try all of the other treatment options we have discussed in this chapter, and if those do not work, and they have the resources, stem cell injections may give them the relief they are seeking from their arthritic pain in their knees, hips, or ankles. But just remember, there are no guarantees. [2,3]

Surgery

When all else fails, yes, there are surgical options that can give you significant relief from your arthritic joint pain. Ranging from minimally invasive arthroscopic surgery to take out a damaged or torn meniscus or to remove loose, articular cartilage to a total knee replacement, surgery can also be a game changer and keep you active and going for many years. I always tell my patients that we will try many of these conservative, nonsurgical options first before considering surgery, but if surgery is necessary, it can make a huge difference in your quality of life at any age. When contemplating surgery, always have a complete understanding with your surgeon what your goals are and what you would like to get out of the surgery, whether it is going back to jogging or skiing or just being able to take a long walk with your spouse. Having realistic expectations is key to having a successful outcome. With new surgical techniques and new surgical materials, surgery can be a very good option for some, so be open to it if all of these other measures fail.

Conclusion

We have covered a lot of material in this chapter, and I hope it has been very useful. "Empowered aging" in this exciting era of new medical advances has the ability to keep us all active no matter what age we are. It starts with the basics: a good diet, watching your weight, a sensible exercise program combined with strengthening and flexibility that will keep those joints happy and healthy. The exciting world of biologics with the use of platelet rich plasma (PRP) and stem cells have the possibility of transforming our lives; but remember, there is still much research to be done before we know for sure how to use these exciting new treatment methods. In the meantime, by sticking to the basics, most of us will do just fine and stay active much longer than any generation before us.

References

Kajikawa Y, Morihara T, Sakamoto H, Matsuda K, Oshima Y, Yoshida A, Nagae M, Arai Y, Kawata M, Kubo T. Platelet-rich plasma enhances the initial mobilization of circulation-derived cells for tendon healing.

Riboh JC, Saltzman BM, Yanke AB, Cole BJ. Human Amniotic membrane-derived products in sports medicine: Basic Science, early results, and potential clinical applications. Am J Sports Med 2015: 1-11

Parolini O, Alviano F, Bagnara GP, et al. Concise review: Isolation and characterization of cells from human term placenta: Outcome of the First International Workshop on Placenta Derived Stem Cells. Stem Cells 2008: 26:300-311

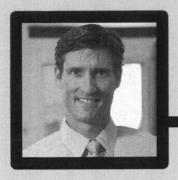

DR. DOMINIQUE M. SCOTT has had over fifty years of family experience and over twenty years of clinical experience in the area of natural health and wellness. Both his parents prioritized natural health in his upbringing, and his father, Dr. Donald R. Scott, was a very successful chiropractic doctor. Dominique has followed in his father's footsteps.

He grew up in Orange County, CA, and attended the University of San Diego as an undergraduate where he completed his Bachelor's Degree and the pre-requisite courses to enter the Doctor of Chiropractic (DC) program at Life University in Marietta, GA. "Dr. Dom" as he is often called, owns and operates a family and sports healthcare practice in Redondo Beach, CA, as well as doing fieldwork as an onsite sports chiropractor for numerous events in junior to pro athletics. In his practice, Dr. Dom, covers health improvement, body performance, and longevity, and has clients who span in age from newborn to ninety. He also teaches these and other topics to sports teams and clubs as well as to other doctors. Dr. Dom is currently developing the performance and prevention content to support the athletes in the AVPFirst junior beach volleyball programs nationwide.

CHAPTER 8

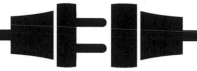

Cross Training for Life—Properties of Movement in Motion

By **DOMINIQUE M. SCOTT, DC**

In my practice, meeting with numerous individuals and families has helped me learn from real-life experiences the connections between aging—particularly what people tend to call "getting old"—and various functions of the human body. In a typical session, I review and discuss a patient's recent and past health and lifestyle history as this is still considered the largest contributor to making a proper diagnosis. Time and again during this consultation, which is the standard process of doctoring, my clients will discuss their chief complaint, go on to list their other chief complaints, and then often even list additional changes in their overall health and life, concluding with a statement like, "It sucks getting old."

Most of the time, these listed complaints include loss of motion—a loss of the way they used to be able to move, and thereby do what they could do at a certain level, or the ability to move without any pain or sign of injury. So they move less, or less comfortably, and therefore cannot do many of the things they used to do, and this is considered standard; it is what many people think of as "getting old." I also know many people who continue their activities, hobbies, or sports a lot longer than others.

Are we destined to lose movement? What do we know about the role of motion and movement for the body as it applies to health, vitality, and longevity?

Movement of and within the human body is a vital mechanism. Movement, or motion, has an essential role from the level of cell to cell interaction, to vital roles in larger tissues, organs, glands, and systems. Moving parts within the body—such as joints, muscles, and vessels—have a vital communication loop with the brain which is activated in large part when motion occurs in those areas.

Looking at the conception of human life, the union of a sperm cell and ovum, it has been observed that one of the first features of this one new cell that was united from two cells is that it begins to move. Movement, motion, is key. It is movement of the lower-leg muscles that serves as a pump to bring the vital blood back up to the heart where cardiac muscle motion cycles the blood with vital nourishment through the body again and again. Motion is used in neurological rehabilitation to stimulate brain nerve pathways that loop from the brain to every muscle and joint in an effort to reignite the ability to move an extremity after a stroke or other brain-body "disconnect" issues.

Conversely, loss of motion, or alterations in motion, results in a loss of efficiency of the involved body parts that were designed to harmonize through movement, including alteration of the brain-to-body loop. For example, the orthopedic method for casting fractures has evolved to shorten the period of time as much as possible that the affected limb is in a hard cast; the idea is to immobilize smaller regions for less time. This change in approach followed the increasing understanding of how crucial motion is for many body processes, including healing. For example, it was discovered that longer periods of immobilization lengthened the time it took for complete recovery and the return of original function.

In these and many other techniques for health, healing, and well-being, motion is recognized as a valuable ingredient for healing and repair. Let these few examples pique our interest as to why movement contributes such vitality in these and many other physiological areas. Let us also investigate further how the vitality of motion in the body can be used proactively for our own healing, performance, prevention of injury, and longevity.

Roots of the Motion Principle

The development of the vast human physiology which stems from movement starts in the earliest moments of life and is a major influence on our body. That initially conceived human life at the cellular level begins moving and is then followed by replication-recreating itself, many times over. This is followed by another incredible cellular change called specialization where the numerous replicated cells move apart to become specialized into the embryo and the embryo life-support components, all now interacting and growing through movement of fluids. As the in utero fetus grows into a baby, many doctors chart the number and frequency of its movements throughout the pregnancy.

Once born, movements and motion are at work in every level of the body. There are movements which are inborn and automatic that are for survival of the new born called reflexes which are part of our brain-body connections. Some of these initial reflexive movements include grasping with hands when the palm is touched, moving toward the breast to eat, swallowing when the roof of the mouth is touched, and extending and contracting the neck and limbs when startled. These reflexive motions promote strength and development of the neuro-musculo-skeletal system, and thereby the ability to make intentional motions, such as looking and turning of the head, reaching with the limbs, rolling over, sitting up, and eventually crawling and walking. The crawling—technically called the "cross-crawl pattern"—that babies do before they walk actually contributes significantly to the development of numerous neurological pathways throughout the body. Yes, brain-body communication develops and is enhanced by the proper motions of crawling.

Most of Us are "Feeling" Oriented

In this case, I'm referring to physical feeling like when a person wakes up with soreness or feels a pain during or after a workout or household chores. These types of sensations and feelings certainly contribute some useful information about what our body has experienced; however, I find most people interpret these feelings incorrectly. In patient consultations—and quite often when hearing people casually discussing their lifestyle issues and adding their own self-diagnoses—most of them conclude that since what they feel—for example, pain or tightness—is localized near a muscle, "X marks the spot," that their sensation area IS the problem. This misconception does not take into account the multiple connections of body parts and structures interacting with their pain area which may actually be causing the problem. Most often, I find the sensation in the area of person's complaint is usually caused by an underlying problem that is affecting the painful location. In many cases, the underlying structural or mechanical problem has been increasing stress to its connecting parts and over time has finally reached the point of eliciting feeling or even initiating a more substantial injury. Often these feelings or symptoms are described as a tightness, soreness, tension, achiness, or spasm. These descriptions will usually be given names or a diagnosis, such as a strain, sprain, muscle spasm, or trigger point. Unfortunately, the diagnosis also tends to cut off the patient's search for what is really happening with his or her body for it to have arrived at this condition and thus what can be done to enable it to feel better through healing correctly. The point behind these scenarios is that the same motion and movement factors that contribute to certain areas of growth, development, brain-body communication and healing also serve a proactive-health role when we utilize motion and movement in our lives regularly for recovery, better body performance and longevity. But these opportunities are too often overlooked if we only pay attention to the feeling or the symptom.

The Body Is always Training

Here we are discussing "training" in the sense of learning, practicing, or developing, like an athlete trains for a sport or a musician trains for a special performance. When training of the body is planned for progressively improving outcomes—as in those previously mentioned applications—the training result is tied to repetitions, or refinements, or repetition of the right actions. Training the body physically for athletics or fitness has a significant basis in motion and movement and reaps greater benefits when the movements are efficiently coordinated toward an end goal of our choosing. Essentially, these applications of training through movement are a process of developing efficiency and strength in our physiology and our abilities—changes in what we can do with our bodies and how the body performs these actions.

Here is the key, though: The body is always training. Even when we are not in a planned process to improve our body performance for a sport or fitness or optimal health, the body is still, always, training. Our body is training in whatever it is that we do most often with it. The simplified law of training our human selves is repetition over time, and it results in changes. We must be mindful that this process is at work whether we choose the inputs that are repeated or not, and therefore we can purposefully direct the changes toward our health and fitness goals for life, or the changes will, by default, go toward a different, and less desirable, end result.

The Concept: "It's All Part of Getting Old"

I will start by clarifying that I understand that there are fundamental changes that occur in our bodies as we live longer, and they include human functions not working the same way they did in earlier years. The part I am addressing here is that there are many contributing factors as to whether we grow and age at an optimal level of function or not. Our bodies have an amazing built-in capacity to repair and renew and live at a high level of health and vitality. I find these capacities are not commonly tapped into proactively. In some cases, I do find people who are working on including health-revitalizing routines as a priority, but they often only began after they had a significant health crisis. This is a help in their recovery and future well-being; however, if we all gave priority to these health and vitality capacities in a proactive and wellness approach…well, a higher level of health and life would be part of the results. So, let's take a new perspective and hopefully some related, action steps toward this purpose of tapping into our capacities for optimal health and body performance throughout the years (and you can begin right now, at whatever age).

In clinic consultations with patients, most people discuss getting older with me from their point of view that everything can be blamed on their age. Two important considerations should be addressed for perspective's sake when looking at aging. One consideration is that the biggest factor for our "getting old" is how the years have been spent. This circles back to our earlier description of how the body is always training. If we did not select to routinely train our bodies for fitness or health and performance or longevity, the body trained in whatever we did most often. (Let me interject here and add that I believe it's never too late to start and make a positive impact on our bodies because of the innate powers of the body to heal and thrive with whatever motion you currently have or may not have). If we did not put much priority on how our body spent its time over the years, and the greatest repetitious time periods were spent dedicated to a career, we thereby trained a "career-functioning" body. Let me explain.

In most cases, the common (career-trained) denominator and the longest hours of body positioning (and patterning) was/is the seated position, or for some, repetitive standing or bending. Examples include commuting in a car or other seat; and then sitting at your work-place seat, perhaps behind a desk; then after work, maybe some time relaxing at home or spending some computer time also sitting; even at the gym, perhaps we bike (there's that bike seat) and even do seated weight machines. See the possibilities of the seated-culture effect?

So, once you recognize this pattern, the solution is that now that your priority is fitness and movement, target specific locations where you can put yourself in motion for the purpose of undoing the seat effects on the body. Perhaps you have completed your desk or car-bound career time and have spent many years, even decades, unknowingly repeating patterns in positions that lacked motion. The attention for restoring and a renewed level of motion will be to focus on moving joints of the body in order to open the door for all the body performance, function, and longevity benefits that come with optimal motion of the joints. Otherwise, if you are still in some level of career-mode, from full-time to part-time or consulting level, it behooves you to similarly focus on undoing the seated effects on your body mechanics along with your fitness steps. In this case, some of your joint-motion-focused action plan is to provide recovery from the week in, week out repeated positions and prepare your body for fitness and other life activities that are safer and more effective for you. Also, you may be targeting some long-term restoration of mobility and joint motion from the first three, four, or five decades of your seated lifestyle (e.g., school and work).

Begin with the Spine in Mind; Your Body Does

The spine is essentially the body's mechanical frame. The spine is coupled intimately with the sacrum and pelvis, and from these central framework components they link to the rest of our skeletal mechanics, being the extremities. The mechanical structures are overlayed and interconnected with the muscle system.

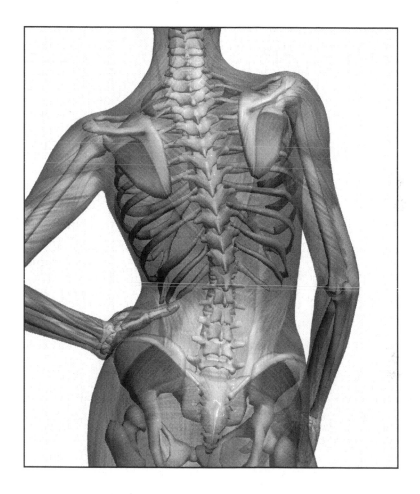

This image reminds us that although our muscles are much easier to feel and even to work on such as with exercise, massage or stretching, that behind the muscles ability to perform their jobs, the ability of the joints to move as designed carry a significant influence. This image reminds us of the numerous muscles anchoring to the spine and sacrum.

All of our moving joints have an ideal designed range of motion, if they lose their ideal range of motion their workload is passed on other joints and also increase stress to muscles, tendons and ligaments. As with other structures, like a building or car for example, if the central frame is off balance, out of position, or if the should-be-moving structures don't move correctly or at all, all other parts are impacted. Therefore in the body, spinal-joint mobility and positioning are primary influences the ability to move efficiently throughout the body. Furthermore, the spinal column has the unique role of housing the spinal cord and exiting nerve roots, which are the information superhighways for a vast amount of our body functions every second of our lives. The spine is the conduit of our brain-to-body and body-to-brain communication and that communication is impacted by good or bad spinal-joint motion and function. (This is a HUGE health factor, if you did not catch that). The spinal cord and its communications with all our body systems never rests, even when we sleep, and yet we do little or nothing to support the health of its interconnected protection system, the spine.

In summary, profound health influences and benefits are available to us by including—in fact, prioritizing—methods to maintain healthy motions of our joints, starting with the spinal joints outward to all the extremities. The bonus of giving focused attention to healthy joint motion is that the muscles come along for the ride; that is, when we work on maintaining proper joint motion, the muscles get the benefit of moving efficiently, as well, similar to what is done nowadays and is called dynamic stretching. As well, the proper mobility and positioning of the spinal column is a major influence of the brain-nerve-body communication.

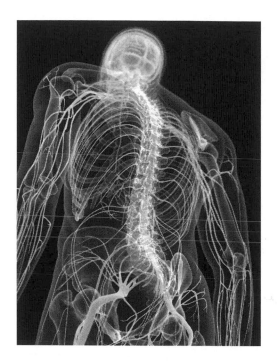

In this photo the brain, spinal cord and main nerve network is imaged to remind us that within the spine is the spinal cord transmitting hundreds or trillions of brain messages to run our body every second. Altered spine motion or position alter the brain-body messaging.

Joint Motion...The Game Changers

When people cannot move the way they used to and therefore drop hobbies, sports, or other activities that require motion, it is predominantly loss of joint motion that is the game-changer. The system of joints—from the vertebra at the spine and throughout our body—are similar to a system of pulleys, like the rigging for sailing or the rigging for cranes and other movable support systems. The muscle groups are similar to the ropes or cables that pull or push the pulleys (or joints in our bodies) and together make the movement of the body parts possible.

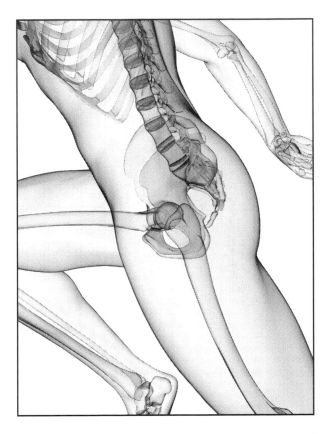

The repetitive positions and stresses to the same areas of our bodies over time alter the ability of joints to move; therefore, the joints, our pulleys, tighten or fixate or move less and change the workload into the muscles significantly. This is compensated for throughout the skeleton and muscles. We usually "feel" the load in the muscles, and it often feels good and even relieves this feeling of muscle load to work on the muscles by stretching or massage or foam-rolling, but this only minimally helps problematic joint function. In this process, the muscle tension or ache will typically reoccur since the altered workload from the faulty joint motion has not been improved and continues the wear and tear on the joint and to the compensating joints and muscle groups. Usually, this further compounds and creates greater strain on the same or nearby joints and causes these parts to be more prone to injury.

So to be clear, when we are doing muscle stretching or releasing techniques, we are only minimally and perhaps not at all counteracting the life effects on the joints. Injuries people experience in this day and age that affect what they can and cannot do lifestyle-wise most often involve a joint; just think about it. The knees that wear out; the shoulders, hips, discs that have herniations or degenerate; these still develop even when people are pretty good with doing massage, stretching and exercising. This is because our awareness of our joint health and function typically does not get our attention until it is too late. There are many levels of small changes in joint functions that compound over time as we get older and progress to the loss of joint motion and related joint or muscle injury or weakness or joint degeneration. Simply stated, there is a huge void in our awareness of how to support the health of our body mechanics with a focus on joint motion first and foremost. When this level of our body systems IS cared for, whole-body performance and longevity are positively impacted because of the vast neuro-mechanical integration of our systems.

Focus Here, Benefit on Many Levels

In clinical practice and life in general, I have observed that it's loss of motion—loss of movements our bodies once performed—that is the change that most people complain about when they say they are "getting old." From my experience, I see that most of us need a greater awareness of how we are and are not using our available body movements. Specifically, we should note which positions our joints are in most often and the directions and ranges of motion we seldom use. Once we gain this awareness, we can apply an approach that will be restorative and improve the performance of our neuro-mechanical well-being.

I call this approach diverse constructive movement. When you break down this phrase, diverse constructive movement, each part is necessary to create a positive outcome. Let's start with the word movement and define the phrase in reverse. (I use the word motion interchangeably with movement.) So the action step is we need to move. When we choose our motion or movement, it is important for each of us to be able to visualize the skeleton and the joints to some degree. Even without detailed study of the body, we can use our basic knowledge of the skeleton and picture the action our joints undergo versus the role of our muscles.

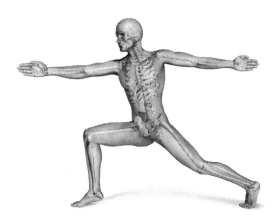

Now, let's add in the priority of routinely moving the joints through the variety of ranges they are naturally designed to move through; that is how we make this action step diverse.

Further defining this approach, let us cover the word constructive. We need to self-evaluate our methods of moving our joints and ask if what we are putting them through is helpful for the body and its parts and not hurtful. The two main factors I recommend we consider is how underused a certain joint motion is and also how overused this motion might be. (If it's already overused in your lifestyle, it's not diverse; if the motion is seldom done, but when we do perform it, we do it too hard or too fast or with too much exertion, it is not constructive.) For example, some men ranging in age from their thirties to their fifties tell me their workout is playing hoops with the guys on weekends. They work all week, forty-plus hours seated in cars, meetings, computers, and then to "work out," they perform (very) diverse movements playing basketball. Is that constructive? No. With a neuromusculoskeletal program of sitting all week for work, the diverse but fast and high-impact motions of basketball are trauma for their joints and associated tissues. If you have or had a lot of sitting hours per week and want to include a sport in your fitness, you need to spend focused attention to preparing the joints gently and constructively for the ranges of motion included in your sport. I recommend you go through standard skills of your sport in very slow motion and while performing them you assess your posture, position of your head, core and legs as well as what muscles and joints feel like they are doing the work. Perform sets of 10 in very slow motion with this acute focus on your body as described above. Then perform a few more sets of 10 slightly faster each time, attempting to hold the form that came with the attention you had on your body at the slow motion version.

In addition, you accrue performance and longevity benefits from including a recovery process from your sport or workouts. Recovery should also include diverse constructive motions of the joints; and remember, when you move the joints, the muscles come along for the ride. Therefore, the muscles have a dynamic warm-up or warm-down, too. For people who are not playing a sport or those not even "working-out," you also gain huge life benefits by incorporating this approach.

Whatever it is you do, and whatever you love to do, having your body there for you for your later years, capable and feeling good, is obviously your goal. I teach the same things to my nonathletic clients because life without attention to the optimal function of your body will likely take some bad turns which were preventable. We teach that everyone, athletic or fit person or not, needs to "cross train for life." This concept arose from the realization that there are better performance results and reduced injury for athletes, when they include diversity in their training plans. The prior concept was that the athlete spent all or a great majority of their training time only on the speed and power gains that directly applied to their sport movements.

The "cross" in cross-training stands for diversify or mix-up your "training". Where training, as explained earlier, is whatever motions (or lacks-of motion) or positions that our lifestyle tends to repeat most often. Living life as a parent, career-focused person, grandparent, and so on, whichever is our role it comes with its own common and repeating demands and stresses on our human structure. Yes we should continue to "train" in cardio and muscle fitness, but if we do not apply the "diverse-constructive-movement" plan to "cross-train" our joints we are undermining all our other fitness efforts. To meet life proactively, and maximize our innate capacity for repair and revitalizing, we should include routinely scheduled joint-focused motions and movements as a primary ingredient of cross-training for life...your life!

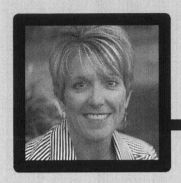

VICTORIA DUPUY has always had a passion for life, love, and learning. In 2013, her life took an unexpected tragic turn when her husband Dean died suddenly of a heart attack at the age of forty-six. Dean led a very active lifestyle and certainly did not fit the profile of someone who was at risk for a heart attack. Upon Dean's death, Victoria immersed herself in learning all she could about heart disease, early detection, and who really is at risk. Through sharing her newly found knowledge and personal experience with friends, family, and the community, Victoria quickly became aware that there were many, many other people with experiences just like hers. This awareness, combined with Victoria's desire to prevent others from experiencing the terrible loss that she and her family went through, was her incentive to found No More Broken Hearts; because for Victoria, every single heart matters.
In the four years since Victoria founded No More Broken Hearts, numerous articles about this unique nonprofit organization have been published in the *San Jose Mercury News*, multiple community newspapers in the Bay area, *M Magazine*, *Bay Area Building Management Resource Guide*, *Los Gatos Living*, and *Saratoga Living*. Victoria is a frequent guest speaker for numerous local and national organizations and has been featured on local Bay area and national radio programs. For Victoria, *the view is worth the climb*, and she will continue to raise awareness and stand for patients' rights until the medical establishment views lives as more important than money.

CHAPTER 9

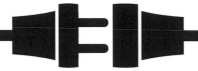

Detecting Silent Heart Disease

By **VICTORIA DUPUY**

On September 29, 2013, my husband, Dean Dupuy, died suddenly of a heart attack at the age of forty-six with no warning at all. He had no health risks, no family history of heart disease, was not overweight, and never smoked a day in his life. He was physically active, biking, running, and playing ice hockey. He had passed his annual physical months before and was told he was in excellent health. But when he died, it was revealed that although he fit the image of someone not at risk, he actually was at risk and had a life-threating level of plaque in his arteries that had ruptured. After twenty-two years of building a life together, it was gone.

I called his doctor a few days later who informed me, "We just don't test patients that are at low risk. It's not like getting a mammogram or a colonoscopy." The Framingham Risk Predictor Scale [1] that was developed back in the fifties is an algorithm that is used based upon a series of questions to determine cardiovascular risk over the next ten years. While many years ago, this was a very useful way in determining risk; it is not very useful today, especially in the world of technology we are in. It is guessing someone's heart health – not testing someone's heart health. For example, if there was a pipe that was in water and we wanted to know if there is corrosion INSIDE the pipe – would we test the water or would we look inside the pipe? It's really the same analogy. Our doctor does not decide what our risk of breast cancer or colon cancer is by looking at us. They refer us for mammogram and colonoscopies to look inside for the cancer. That is where my journey started. I spent weeks learning everything I could about heart disease, who really is at risk, and if there were preventative screenings like mammograms and colonoscopies that if offered could prevent something like this.

During this journey, I discovered that there is a simple, non-invasive test called a Coronary Artery Calcium Scan (aka CACS; the mammogram of the heart and/or heart scan) that identifies heart disease at it earliest stages so it can be managed, treated, monitored, and in some cases, reversed (mostly through aggressive diet changes). This preventative screening has been around for over twenty years and yet it still is not mainstream in our annual physicals even though there are thousands of studies and clinical trials attesting to its validity. While there are other cardiac screenings recommended should you be at risk based upon the Framingham Risk Predicator Scale, CACS is not one of them. The "go to" preventative screening recommended is a Stress Test" or an Echocardiogram. While both of these tests are valuable in determining if there are any blockages in the artery, they do not determine or identify plaque burden BEFORE it becomes a blockage in the artery. I started connecting with cardiologists around the United States that use this CACS regularly in their practice to prevent patients from having heart attacks and confirmed what I was learning. As a matter of fact, several indicated that over half of the heart attacks that occur are preventable with early detection. I still struggled with understanding this—mammograms save lives, colonoscopies save lives—why are we not doing heart scans of the most important organ in our body?

As I went out into my community with this knowledge, I learned that my story was not that unique. Everyone I spoke to knew someone or knew someone who knew someone who had had a heart attack who did not fit the image of someone at risk. That was the moment for me when I understood that there was a problem; that most of the public was completely unaware of this test. This became a game changer for me and know deep in my heart and soul that I need to try and change this. Every minute of every day there is another unexpected heart attack, and there are far too many broken hearts left behind to cope. According to the Center for Disease Control and Prevention, *"about 610,000 people die of heart disease every year in the United States – that's 1 in 4 deaths. Heart Disease is the leading cause of death of both men and women. Every year approximately 735,000 American's have heart attacks; of these 525,000 are first heart attacks and 210,000 happen in people that already had a heart attack* [2]*."*

No More Broken Hearts is a California non-profit that was created in 2014 to provide education and raise awareness about Coronary Artery Calcium Scans (CACS) and how this simple test can identify heart disease early before a heart attack happens. It was created to empower the public to educate themselves and talk to their doctors whether you have "risk factors" or not, no matter how healthy you feel, because heart disease does impact the most unusual suspects. Nomorebrokenhearts.info/resources and YouTube have hundreds of studies and videos about the subject. If your doctor feels you aren't at risk and that you don't need a CACS, then get a new doctor. Men over the age of forty and women over the age of fifty-five (or earlier depending on when menopause occurs) should be getting their hearts checked out. You get a mammogram or a PSA test and a colonoscopy; add this test to your list. Be sure to get a CACS, too. If you don't want to do it for yourself, then do it for all the hearts that will be left behind.

Resources

DAWBER, T.R., MOORE, F.E., and MANN, G.V., 1957. Coronary heart disease in the Framingham Study. American Journal of Public Health, 47, 4-24.

CDC, NCHS. Underlying Cause of Death 1999-2013 on CDC WONDER Online Database, released 2015. Data are from the Multiple Cause of Death Files, 1999-2013, as compiled from data provided by the 57 vital statistics jurisdictions through the Vital Statistics Cooperative Program. Accessed Feb. 3, 2015

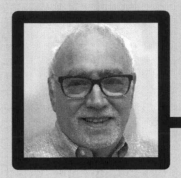

DR. ROBERT A WEIL, sports podiatrist, has treated many of the world's premier athletes from all types of sports and is the host of "The Sports Doctor™" Radio Show. The show is featured on Starcom Radio Network, UK Health Radio & Sports 4 Fanz Radio. Dr. Bob was formerly on HealthyLife.Net Radio and was also on WDCB public radio in Chicago for over 20 years. He has written for many newspapers & magazines and is a frequent guest on many other networks. Dr. Bob's articles & past shows are available on his website at: sportsdoctorradio. com

CHAPTER 10

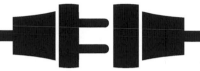

Aging—It's a Balancing Act

By **DR. ROBERT A WEIL**

Whether you are a great athlete or a great-grand-mother, balance is a very important ingredient. Both examples show the importance of balance in everyday life or high-performance athletes. The older we get, the more important it becomes!

One of the largest segments of our population, older senior citizens, face the challenges of fall prevention. Doctors and physical therapists are paying lots of attention to this. In podiatry, this is a hot topic that takes into account the importance of proper shoes, exercise, and orthotics, which are all important parts of programs to prevent falls.

Let's take a look at balance—what it is, what its components are—and the practical applications that can help you improving it.

The term *proprioception* means "sense of self." Proprioceptive *signals* from the joints, muscles, tendons, and skin are essential for movement. These signals give the brain information about the position of the body and limbs in space at any given time. The loss of these signals may affect the control of muscle tone, disrupt reflexes, and severely impair voluntary movement.

Imagine the dancer gliding across the room, not looking where she is going, or someone going down a flight of stairs at night without the lights on without falling. Or, stand on one foot and close your eyes. All are examples of these proprioceptive abilities. We are able to go through daily activities that require all types of body movements without giving it much attention.

A key point I'd like to emphasize is that we can improve our proprioception and balance regardless of what activity we're doing. Weakness in this balance ability as we get older often brings it to our attention. Trying to improve performance in sports at all levels also makes balance improvement front and center.

Senior citizens and older people are quite concerned about falling and falling prevention. People want to keep active, keep walking, and enhance their fitness. I've seen proprioceptive and balance exercises help this population immensely.

I like to call the category of proprioceptive and balance exercises "instability training." I developed this term and definition along with renowned kinesiotherapist Bob Gajda with whom I treated some of the world's greatest athletes over the past three decades. Equipment like minitrampolines, balance boards, and balance beams were typically used to purposely "create imbalance" and thus demand active stabilizer muscles to work. Stabilizer muscles work to stabilize the body and its extremities during multi-plane movements. Think of these exercises as working the stabilizer muscles and tendons surrounding and supporting the feet and ankles, knees, hips, and back. The postural core muscles, which act as a corset holding you together rather than moving your trunk, also become active. All these areas are important for stability and structural integrity.

Your foot type and mechanics along with your body type also can play a role in balance as you get older. Flat feet, high arches, differences in leg length, knock knees, and bowed legs are all examples of factors that affect our balance. I've often prescribed orthotics or custom foot inserts for my older patients as balance becomes more of an issue.

Proper shoes also are very important, and support on the ground is key. Wearing slip-on shoes, flip-flops, or loose, non-supportive sandals are good examples of what *not* to wear. Good walking shoes, with proper support, are the way to go. Often, orthotics are used to replace the insole in the shoes for optimum foot, ankle, and lower-leg alignment. Everyone is familiar with the song, "The foot bone is connected to the ankle bone, the ankle bone is connected to the knee bone," and so on. Paying attention to the function of the feet and their effect on all areas above them is important when it comes to the challenges of balance from superstars to grandmas!

In summary, balance is often a concern, especially as we age. Safety in this area and being proactive in the prevention of problems makes great sense. Combining exercise for stability and balance along with attention to foot and body structure is smart.

Be aware that, as we get older, our body changes; our muscles might not be as flexible, strong, or supple, and our joints might be stiffer. All these factors can affect our balance.

Whatever our age, level of fitness, or activity, keep in mind that *balance is the key*.

PART 3

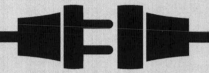

Integrative, Holistic and Natural Approaches to Aging

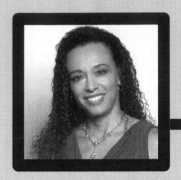

DR. MYLAINE RIOBE is double board certified in Integrative Medicine and OB-GYN and has over sixteen years of experience. Dr. Riobe's undergraduate studies were completed at Columbia University in New York City where she grew up. She obtained her medical degree at New York Medical College and completed her residency in Obstetrics and Gynecology at Medical College of Pennsylvania and the University of South Carolina. There she learned conventional medical practices that she used for four years. She quickly grew frustrated with the cookie-cutter medicine that she had learned.

This led her to the study of traditional Chinese medicine and integrative medicine over the following eight years. She completed her studies at the Academy of Pain Research, a University of California, Irvine-affiliated institution; the University of Miami; and the American Academy of Anti-Aging Medicine. She obtained her board certification in the newly recognized field of Integrative Medicine in 2017.

As a woman and a mom, she knows firsthand how we can all be consumed by a hectic lifestyle. Therefore, she practices what she preaches by living an active, balanced lifestyle that includes healthy eating and exercise.

CHAPTER 11

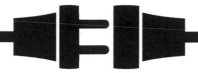

Integrative Medicine: The Missing Link to Successful Aging

By **MYLAINE RIOBE, MD**

ost people think of aging as the progression of time since birth. While that seems logical enough, it's fundamentally wrong. We often see those people that, although they get older, never seem to age. What's their secret? We often attribute it to good genes...or is it? Despite our genes, our levels of disease have been on the rise. Cancer is about to surpass heart attacks as the number one killer of American adults. If good genes were the cause of good health, we wouldn't see the escalation of diseases over time that we are witnessing today.

Many Americans, 50 percent of the population, have at least one chronic disease before age eighteen! Our children are getting diseases in their teens that prior generations didn't get until their forties or fifties! This onslaught of disease is shortening our lifespans, and more importantly, eroding our quality of life. For the first time in over two hundred years, our children are not expected to live as long as we do. And our seniors are also suffering the ill effects of our toxic modern lifestyles. Alzheimer dementia is on the rise, too. Before we allow all this doom and gloom to take hold, take heart! There's a solution!

At the Riobe Institute of Integrative Medicine, I've successfully helped people of all ages get and stay healthy. I'll share with you the 5 Pillars of great health that we use at the Riobe Institute. Because we've lost touch with our bodies and how they actually function, we've also lost our health. *Integrative medicine* is a holistic system of medicine drastically different from our conventional, American, allopathic system of medicine. Our American allopathic system diagnoses and treats diseases thereby masking the symptoms of disease. While this is critical for life threatening conditions, it's not as useful for prevention of disease. *Integrative medicine* seeks the causes of symptoms and conditions from their roots and treats them with natural alternatives for a safer path to wellness and prevention. Aging gracefully and maintaining independence during our golden years is of paramount importance, and most seniors don't get the advice they really need from their conventional medical doctors. In this chapter, I'll share the 5 Pillars to good health that I share with my patients.

Pillar 1: Getting Old Takes Guts!

We often hear the mantra, "You are what you eat!" While that's true most of the time, we're finding out it's a little deeper than that. I have many patients who come to see me because they eat healthy and still get sick. If we are what we eat, why isn't it enough to stay healthy by eating healthy?

It boils down to this: It doesn't matter what we eat if the very system that needs to break food down—absorb it so our cells can use it for fuel—isn't working! Because the gut is exposed to the environment, it's exposed to a lot of toxins and "bad" bacteria that wreak havoc with its function. Many Americans have symptoms directly related to the gut, such as bloating, gas, belching, nausea, constipation, loose stools, and heartburn. They often take medications to mask the distressing symptoms, but these symptoms are critical to letting you know that the most important system in your body isn't working properly.

The human gut has recently been identified as the most complex ecosystem on planet Earth! This startling discovery came as a result of the government-sponsored Human Microbiome Project that started in 2012. This project aimed to map out the genes of the 100 trillion "good" bacteria (called the *microbiome*) that live in the human gut.

The Human Genome Project of 2004 identified that our human cells contain roughly 20,000 genes that orchestrate body function. This was a real disappointment because we thought that organisms as complex as the human body would contain millions of genes. Basically, after this study, we discovered that the common houseplant had more genes than we did! Big blow to the ego. In contrast, the Human Microbiome Project led to the discovery that the good bacteria, or microbiome, houses 3.4 million genes! In other words, 90 percent of our body function relies on little bugs we can't even see that live in our guts and on our skin. Ancient Chinese physicians knew about the importance of gut function over 3,500 years ago—they called it "spleen qi" (pronounced *chee*). In fact, there were and still are entire schools in Chinese medicine dedicated to the study of the energy system called "spleen."

The other key point here is the environment in which these genes live inside the cells determines how they are turned on or off to control body function. So, when we're surrounded by toxins and eat them, too, bad things happen.

The most important step in maintaining good health is to get the gut healthy. Many people think that taking probiotics is the solution, but that's a small part of keeping the gut healthy. Probiotics are basically the "good bugs" in a capsule. A high-quality probiotic is good, but if your gut isn't working properly, that won't be enough.

The four steps to recovering proper gut function are the following:

1. Obtain a functional gut study to determine if you have sufficient enzyme production and absorption of nutrients, infections, leaky gut membranes, and more. An integrative doctor can assist you in obtaining these tests and provide a proper assessment and interpretation of the results once he or she knows your medical history and symptoms. We perform functional gut studies at the Riobe Institute as a cornerstone for the majority of our patients. You don't have to be seen in the office to obtain great results from taking this test.

2. If you are diagnosed with a gut infection, it's critical to get it treated immediately and successfully. Conventional testing often misses infections in the gut, so functional gut studies are critical for accurate results. Infections can be treated

with antibiotics or other natural antimicrobials. Treating gut infections can be tricky because infectious bacteria have developed defense mechanisms that make it hard to get rid of them. An expert in eradicating these infections can properly guide you.

3. The best diet in the world will not overcome an infection in the gut or a leaky gut. It's critical to know the status of the gut and have a step-by-step guide to treating any dysfunction. While it seems like a lot to do, it pays huge dividends in the end. Good gut function can ward off dementia, depression, anxiety, and loss of muscle mass and bone density.

4. Remember that you can have no gut symptoms at all and still have significant malabsorption of nutrients or an infection. I have countless patients who had no symptoms but were getting sick, and it all boiled down to their gut function!

Having said that, there are some "do-it-yourself" tricks that can help. Tips for gut health include the following:

1. Eat a broad and varied diet. Variety is the spice of life especially with food choices!

2. Increase fermented foods in the diet. Fermented foods feed the good bacteria that live in the gut to help them thrive. Examples of traditional fermented foods are kimchi, kefir, miso, sourdough, tepa, and kombucha.

3. High-dose garlic helps break down the protective barriers of the "bad" bacteria to make them more susceptible to the body's natural defenses.

4. Consider guar gum, a soluble fiber that is fermented or metabolized by good bacteria and helps seal a leaky gut.

5. Assuring proper zinc levels helps boost the immune system and also improves gut permeability (that is, a leaky gut).

6. Glutamine is an amino acid that is the primary energy source for the cells of the gut.

7. Iron supplementation, if diagnosed as deficient, helps boost immunity and improves gut permeability.

8. Probiotics have been shown to have many health benefits including boosting immunity and repairing the gut barrier lining to improve gut permeability.

9. Colostrum, naturally found in human breast milk, can be found in supplements also containing immune factors IgG and lactoferrin.

10. Omega-3 fatty acids such as that found in fish oils have been shown to improve gut barrier function and treat leaky gut.

11. Eat fresh organic fruits and vegetables to maximize fiber, phytonutrients, and flavonoids shown to interact with the cells of the body to improve immunity and heal the gut.

12. Avoid chemically processed foods and artificial substances such as NSAIDs (synthetic anti-inflammatory drugs) that erode the mucous lining of the gut. Many foods contain pesticides that also damage the good bacteria and leave us prone to infection and a leaky gut. Eating organic foods helps lessen the burden of pesticides.

13. Avoid artificial sweeteners as they have been shown to cause disturbances in metabolism through disruption of the gut microbiome. Stevia or honey are considered safe sweeteners. Stevia is relatively calorie-free whereas honey has some calories.

14. *Prebiotics* are foods that remain undigested by the human

gut but can be digested by the good bacteria so they can thrive. Examples are carbohydrates known as "resistive." They include green bananas, green plantains, oatmeal, cooked then cooled white potatoes, cooked then cooled white rice.

Pillar 2: Adrenal Function: Stressing-out Over Getting Old

We could debate all day which system is most abused in the human body: the gut or the adrenal system? It's a close call, for sure. Stress in the twenty-first century is like nothing we've ever seen before as a species. The adrenal system is the stress-handling system responsible for our fight or flight responses to threats. When we evolved as a species, we came with built-in fight or flight mechanisms to help us survive and multiply as a species. When we were threatened by predators, we had instant reactions that increased our heart rate and blood pressure and fed sugar to our muscles to fight or run so we could be safe. Back then, predators either ate us alive or we fled into our caves for safety. Either way, the fight or flight response didn't last long—we were either alive or dead within seconds. It was a brief and basic survival mechanism.

Fast forward forty thousand years, and this same mechanism is alive and well today. The difference now is that this fight or flight mechanism is chronically active. We are exposed to over 180 cancer-causing toxins daily and stressful psychological circumstances such as financial stress, family stress, job-related stress, and more. Deep inside our cells where our body functions take place, there are no eyes and brains to assess threats. So, while we, as an organism, can survey a situation and know we're not immediately threatened, we are still producing stress hormones to help us cope with chronic stress, and these chronic stress hormones go right into our cells!

Our cells are responding as though we're being chased by a bear because they are responding to the chemistry of stress, whether it's chronic or acute. The cells never shut off the fight or flight mechanism until they think the coast is clear, and under chronic stress, that seldom happens. So, our stress mechanisms are always on as if we were driving our cars without ever turning off the engine. Imagine keeping your engine on all day and all night—that would be a catastrophe, yet this is what we do to our cells every day, year after year. It's no wonder our cells malfunction, just as our cars would if we never shut them off.

Cortisol is the hormone produced by the adrenal system in response to chronic stress. Low cortisol is often seen in patients with cancer, heart disease, Alzheimer dementia, and other conditions. Low cortisol results from a very taxed system in someone who has been under chronic stress for years.

Proper treatment of the adrenal system combines a stress-reduction strategy with adequate support. Some tips for successful stress reduction are as follows:

1. Exercise consistently. Moderate exercise is great stress relief. Staying active helps improve circulation, boost metabolism, and mitigate the impact of stress. It's important to warm up with a gentle walk, then stretch the whole body gently before exercising. Be sure to obtain clearance from your physician before starting an exercise regimen.

2. Meditation has been consistently shown with functional brain scanning to reduce the impact of stress, lower blood

pressure, improve memory, and more. The benefits of meditation are well studied and proven. Just as little as twenty minutes a day can make a huge difference. Meditation can be as simple as focusing on feeling the air move in and out of your nostrils. It's important not to chastise yourself for thinking or losing focus. That's why it's called a practice. Losing focus is simply a gentle reminder to refocus. It's always a great idea to study with a master if you have the opportunity. Remember the goal of meditation is not to stop thinking, it's to focus your thinking on your breathing.

3. Testing the adrenal system is possible with saliva testing, which has been shown in studies to be a superior method of testing when compared to doing blood work.[1] Saliva testing is the gold standard for assessing the adrenal system. Typically, samples are obtained just after awakening, at noon, 4 p.m., and at 8 p.m. This curve is matched to what is considered normal, and you can see how you measure up, so to speak. Depending on the interpretation of these results, there are multiple adrenal supplements that can target the particular imbalances you might have in your system. For consistently high cortisol, adaptogens are helpful. Examples are ashwagandha, panax ginseng, bacopa, cordyceps, and others. For low cortisol, adrenal extracts may be more beneficial. For extremely low cortisol such as that found in users of artificial steroids, supplementation with cortisol may be necessary for proper function. For mixed, high- and low-cortisol counts, the combination of adaptogens with licorice may be helpful. It's important to seek help from

a board-certified Integrative Medical Doctor for proper adrenal support.

4. Sleep is a critical stress-reduction mechanism. The body restores itself while we sleep. Sleep deprivation has been associated with just about every disease because if we don't sleep sufficiently, we don't recover and repair our cells, which leads to malfunction. If you have chronically low or low-normal cortisol, it's important to consistently get nine hours of sleep nightly. If you have difficulty sleeping, I recommend a sleep study. Artificial light from computer and TV screens is a common culprit in sleep disorders. Obtaining blue-light-blocking glasses that you wear from dusk until you go to sleep helps block harmful light from these screens that incorrectly signals to the body that it's time to wake up.

Pillar 3: Hormones—Friend or Foe?

In 2004, the Women's Health Initiative Study was released revealing very bad news for users of hormone replacement therapy—specifically, conjugated equine estrogens combined with medroxyprogesterone, a *synthetic* form of hormones given to menopausal women in the United States for over forty years! This study was stopped prematurely due to the alarming increase in breast cancer and strokes observed in the women taking these hormones. The WHI study remains controversial because critics argue that the women studied were older and already had risk factors for stroke and cancer. While this study was and remains controversial, there really is no controversy when you look at a few things.

First, these hormones are *synthetic*. When it comes to body function inside our cells, synthetic is never good! *Synthetic* means that the chemical structure of the hormone or medication is not natural and looks different than what the body is supposed to use for functioning.

Hormones are basically blueprints for body function. Once made in the cells, they circulate throughout the body to where they are needed. Hormones function throughout the entire body, contrary to what we are taught. We often mistakenly believe that the hormones made in the ovaries and testes are only used for reproduction. That couldn't be further from the truth. In fact, estrogen alone has over four hundred functions in the human body, both male and female! Estrogen is responsible for hair growth, vision, skin health, immunity, digestion, breathing, bone and muscle health, reproduction, and much more!

If there is synthetic estrogen in the cells instead of natural estrogen, the body's cells are misguided and don't perform the same functions, and this spells disaster long-term. The hormones used in the WHI study were synthetic, and it's no surprise that they caused more problems than they solved.

The second issue with these hormones is that they are not monitored. When we prescribe hormones in our allopathic system, we prescribe them based on hot flashes or night sweats and other menopausal symptoms. We've learned the hard way that it's not prudent to do this. Symptoms have many possible causes, and many different hormones can be responsible for the symptoms we experience, so knowing which hormones someone needs requires proper testing.

Blood work is not very accurate and doesn't reflect the "functioning" hormones in the body. In fact, the blood stream is a transportation highway and shows us what is in transit from one place to another place, but tells us nothing about the inside of the cells where hormones are active. Cellular-based testing is emerging as a better method of testing based on early studies. Again, using the expertise of a board-certified integrative medical doctor is important for safe and effective hormone balancing.

Stress causes hormone imbalances as a survival mechanism. Our body knows that if we're being chased by predators, it would be wise not to reproduce, so it has built-in mechanisms to suppress hormone production in times of stress. That is why people under stress have higher infertility rates than those not under stress. Under chronic stress, hormones are chronically imbalanced. Getting them back into balance is a cornerstone for maintaining good health.

With all this confusion about hormones, where does one begin? *Bioidentical hormones* have been used in Europe for over forty years, and they have been well studied in Europe for over twenty-five years. Bioidentical hormones have three critical attributes. The first is that they are natural and made of soy or yam. They are engineered to look just like our own hormones, which is why they are called bioidentical. This is the main reason for their safety-they don't look different than our hormones are supposed to look. Lastly, their use is monitored. In other words, the levels of hormone in the body are measured and used in dosing. Studies on bioidentical hormones have consistently shown them to be safer than our US-based hormones. Bioidentical hormones have been shown to reduce the risk of certain cancers, especially breast cancer; to reduce the risk of heart attacks and strokes; as well as reduce the risk of Alzheimer dementia. There have also been longevity and quality-of-life studies that have shown favorable results with bioidentical hormones. [2,3,4]

To be taken safely, you must be tested properly to determine your needs. Once on hormones, your levels inside your cells must be closely monitored to assure the levels are normal and balanced with other hormones.

Lastly, you must have good nutrition to assure those hormones are properly used, metabolized, and eliminated by your cells so that toxic hormone levels don't build up.

Having chronically low hormone levels is dangerous and has been shown to be linked to many diseases of aging such as Alzheimer dementia, heart disease, and more, so hormone balancing should be considered a part of a complete wellness program. There are certain contraindications to hormone replacement therapy, and you should be thoroughly evaluated before beginning a hormone replacement program.

Another common myth is that older people shouldn't be given hormones. This doesn't apply to bioidentical hormones because they are not associated with increased risks of strokes like synthetic hormones are. It's important to start with low doses and slowly increase the dosage level, but only if monitoring warrants it. The goals are to have normal and balanced levels in the cells with the lowest doses possible to achieve those goals.

TIPS FOR HORMONE BALANCE

Because stress directly suppresses hormone balance, it's difficult to keep them naturally balanced without consistently practiced stress-relief techniques such as meditation, exercise, adequate sleep, and excellent nutrition, which we've reviewed in previous sections. It all comes full circle!

Pillar 4. Detoxification—Taking Out the Garbage!

Our cells are constantly active performing our body functions. Every second of our lives, cells are performing billions of chemical reactions. Just like any other place where a lot of work gets done, things tend to get dirty. If the cells don't also include cleaning themselves as part of their function, they quickly begin to malfunction. *Detoxification* is a complex system that occurs in all cells to remove gunk and debris to keep the cells working optimally. These systems require fuel to work—this comes in the form of nutrition. It's critical to eat the right foods that will fuel the detox systems of the cells.

Studies are showing that the average American is exposed to 180-200 different cancer-causing toxins (known as *carcinogens*) daily![5] In fact, many babies today are exposed to these toxins even before birth through the umbilical cord of their mom's womb. Once we're born, this exposure continues daily. It's no wonder that cancer is becoming more common. What a lot of people don't know is that these same toxins don't just cause cancer. They contribute to a lot of aging diseases that erode our quality of life and rob us of our independence. It's critical to maintain detoxification systems in tip-top shape to maintain proper body function. While the liver is widely known as an important detoxification system in the body, it only deals with what ends up in the bloodstream. The gastrointestinal system is responsible for detoxification of anything we consume before it's released into the bloodstream and is now considered the most critical detoxification system in the body! There's that circle again...

The skin is also a detoxification system for anything that is absorbed through our pores. Our skin removes harmful chemicals and defends the body from invaders.

These three systems are responsible for defending the body from toxins, and each and every cell ultimately is responsible for keeping itself clean. Just like all other body functions, detoxification requires a ton of vitamins, minerals, anti-oxidants, amino acids, and hormones to function. We can begin to see how all the systems of the body are *interdependent*; in other words, they rely on each other for their proper function. If one system fails, it puts a significant burden on the others to compensate. We are a unified, seamless whole.

TIPS FOR EFFECTIVE DETOXIFICATION

1. My patients often ask me if they should use a detoxification regimen to remove toxins from the body. As I most often do, I say, "It depends." What does it depend on? It depends on the reserve energy of the body to tolerate the detox regimen. If someone has weak reserves and they do an intensive detoxification protocol, they can make themselves sicker and even more prone to toxin build-up. Forcing the body to detox when it's weak just makes it weaker, so like everything else, balance is the key.

2. A quick way to assess if you might tolerate a detox regimen is to assess how you feel after a moderate to strenuous workout. If you feel pretty wiped out and have difficulty recovering, you're probably not a good candidate for any intensive detoxification protocol, particularly if it's not guided by your doctor. For people who are too weak to

detox, it's more important to fortify the detox mechanisms of the body with really good nutrition.

3. Eating a diet high in green, leafy vegetables is a great way to boost the body's natural detoxification mechanisms. These foods are rich in vitamins, minerals, and antioxidants that fuel the cells' detoxification mechanisms. Raw vegetable juicing can be great, but isn't for everyone. If you do a raw vegetable juicing protocol and don't feel good, try putting those veggies in a warm broth and cooking them instead. This makes it easier to digest and may be better tolerated than the raw vegetables.

4. Supplements that help the detoxification mechanisms are N-acetyl cysteine, CoQ10, milk thistle, B complex vitamins, vitamin C, calcium, magnesium, manganese, and zinc.

Pillar 5: Lifestyle Management: Putting It All Together

I will discuss how planning the day is a cornerstone to empowered aging. Flying by the seat of your pants is fun sometimes, but if we manage our nutrition, exercise, and sleep strategies this way, we often skip the most important parts of our day. Staying healthy requires a healthy paranoia and consistency to follow a solid plan day in and day out. Of course, we all fall off the bandwagon occasionally, but getting back on the bandwagon as soon as possible is the key to success.

Becoming a student of good health is a critical part of managing a lifestyle.

1. Learn to read food labels so you know exactly what's going into your body. Avoid processed foods as much as possible.

2. Eating locally grown, fresh organic fruits and vegetables is a cornerstone of any good plan.

3. If you are a meat or poultry eater, be sure to eat grass-fed, organic meats and poultry. This includes your eggs!

4. Make certain you are obtaining the correct proportions of your macronutrients (proteins, fats, and carbohydrates).

5. Reading your labels or looking up the macronutrient proportions of foods on the Internet is the best way to learn what's going in. There is considerable controversy about the best proportions. A general guideline for sedentary people: 0.5-0.7 grams of protein and 0.5-0.7 grams of carbohydrates per pound of body weight. No more than 30 percent of your calories should come from fats, even the good ones. This adds up to 0.25 grams of fat per pound of body weight on average. Of course, this is not an exact science, so you have to gauge your progress and increase and decrease your proportions until you find your optimal range. Anyone with liver or kidney disease may need to have their proportions further adjusted.

6. If you're actively exercising three to four times a week, you'll need to increase these proportions accordingly. Active exercise requires a lot of protein and a lot of calories, so increasing your protein and carbs is essential to supporting the activity so that you aren't prone to injuries, fatigue, or damage to your metabolism.

A general guideline for moderately active people is 1.0 grams of protein and 1.0 grams of carbohydrates per pound of lean body weight. Again, keep your fats to about 30 percent of your calories, or 0.25 grams of fat per pound of lean body weight.

Many people think that carbohydrates are the enemy, however, this isn't really true. The trick is to consume only what you will burn and not overeat carbohydrates in any one meal. Nutrition is the cornerstone of a healthy lifestyle followed by exercise and sleep!

Exercise guidelines vary, but I'm a big fan of resistance training with such options as Pilates, circuit training, resistance bands, or other options that help maintain muscle mass and bone strength. Our muscles are a direct indication of our metabolism. Our bone is a direct indication of our reserve metabolic energy. These are based in ancient traditional Chinese medicine principles and ring true to this day. Maintaining muscle mass is also an anti-aging strategy because of the preservation of *metabolism*, which is the energy that our body uses to power its functions. The more muscles we have, the more energy we have to power body functions.

I also strongly advise against overexercising, which I believe is just as bad as underexercising. It's critical to have balance. If you're just starting an exercise routine, I strongly recommend the guidance of a certified trainer in resistance training. If you're just starting out, it's normal to feel sore and tired afterward, but you should quickly adapt and feel really good after your activities. If you feel wiped out the next day or find it hard to go about your day, that's a big indicator that the activity is too much, and you should reduce its intensity. Generally, it's good to be active daily with a brisk walk, swim, mild yoga, or bike ride. It's good to have a resistance training regimen you follow consistently three to four times a week. Change it up and don't always do the same thing, or your body will get used to it and the benefits will wane.

Sleep is a critical part of aging gracefully, and seniors are notorious for getting less sleep as they age, partly because of the difficulty in sleeping that many experience. Sleep deprivation has become a part of our culture and is dangerous. Men generally should sleep about seven hours a night. If you have low reserves, such as in the case of adrenal fatigue, you need nine hours. Women in general should obtain about eight hours of sleep with the same recommendations for nine hours in the presence of adrenal fatigue.

Melatonin is an important hormone in sleep regulation. Melatonin is made at night while we sleep and tells the body to "sleep." Chronic sleep deprivation and exposure to artificial light interfere with melatonin production. There are some methods that assist in naturally raising melatonin levels, which avoid the need to take melatonin supplements. Pineapple, mangosteen, and ginger are known to naturally raise melatonin levels. Naturally raising melatonin levels in your body is always better than having to use a supplement.

Minimizing exposure to artificial light is also important, and blue-light-blocker glasses may help if your sleep is interrupted by this light. Properly winding down after your day is a critical part of good sleep habits.

A consistent meditation practice in the evening is a great way to get the brain to quiet down after a busy day. It's generally not a good idea to watch the news or action movies just before bedtime, as this wakes the brain up and puts it in overdrive.

Alcohol is also not a good way to wind down. While alcohol may make you sleepy, it disrupts sleep.

Some nutrients that may help with quieting the brain at night are theanine, which is naturally found in green tea; melatonin, which reduces cortisol levels if they're high; magnesium; and passionflower.

There is also growing concern about devices that emit

electromagnetic fields (EMFs) such as cell phones, computers, TVs, radios, and microwave ovens. EMF is an electromagnetic field emitted from all electric devices. Before being defunded in the 1990s, the Office of Technology Assessment of the US Congress recommended "prudent avoidance" of these devices. The farther away you are from a source of EMF, the better. You can install shielding devices on your computers and cell phones to reduce exposure. Rearranging furniture to be farther away from microwaves, radios, TVs, and so on is also prudent.

Aging in the twenty-first century has become a full-time job. If you thought you were retired, guess again! The key is to become a student of good health. Always maintain a healthy curiosity; engage your physicians, trainers, and consultants to let them know you're serious about maintaining your health and independence. Listen to your body's clues to let you know if you're overdoing it. Work at your own pace, but keep moving forward. If you get stuck, find an integrative medical doctor to assist you.

I wish you many blessings on your journey of wellness.

For more information, visit RiobeIntegrativeMedicine.com

References:

1. Gozansky, WS, et. Al. "Salivary cortisol determined by enzyme immunoassay is preferable to serum total cortisol for assessment of dynamic hypothalamic-pituitary-adrenal axis activity." *Clinical Endocrinology.* 2005; 63:336-341

2. O'Leary, P, et al. "Salivary, but not serum or urinary levels of progesterone are elevated after topical application of progesterone cream to pre- and postmenopausal women." *Clinical Endocrinology.* 2005; 53:615-620

3. Morgantaler, A et al. "Testosterone Therapy and Cardiovascular Risk: Advances and Controversies." Mayo Clinic Proc. February 2015; 90 (2):224–251 18

4. Philip M. Sarrel MD, et al. "The Mortality Toll of Estrogen Avoidance: An Analysis of Excess Deaths Among Hysterectomized Women Aged 50 to 59 Years" American Journal of Public Health, September 2013

5. National Institutes of Health, National Toxicology Program, 14th Report of Carcinogens; 2016

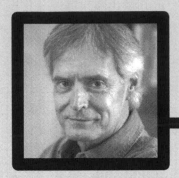

BRANT CORTRIGHT, PHD, is the author of the #1 international Amazon best seller, *The Neurogenesis Diet and Lifestyle: Upgrade Your Brain, Upgrade Your Life.* He is a professor of psychology at the California Institute of Integral Studies in San Francisco. He is also a licensed clinical psychologist with a private practice in neuroscience-informed depth psychotherapy and also has a coaching practice focused on brain health, anxiety, and depression. He is the author of two previous books, *Psychotherapy and Spirit* and *Integral Psychology: Yoga, Growth and Opening the Heart* (both by SUNY Press).

Website: *brantcortright.com*

Facebook: *www.facebook.com/profile.php?id=100009036433305*

Twitter: *twitter.com/brantcortright*

CHAPTER 12

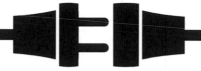

Holistic Brain Health in Aging

By **BRANT CORTRIGHT, PHD**

The brain exists on many levels, which makes healthy aging such a challenge. A *holistic approach* to brain aging allows all levels of our brain to have the optimal stimulation and protection they need for maximum cognitive health. This approach to brain health is spelled out much more fully in my book, *The Neurogenesis Diet and Lifestyle: Upgrade Your Brain, Upgrade Your Life.*

Holistic health claims that only by looking at every level of our being can we find true health. We exist on the physical level (body), the emotional level (heart), the mental level (mind), and the spiritual level (spirit or soul.) The human brain encompasses all four dimensions of our being because we experience everything through our brain.

To live our life at our highest potential, we need our brain to operate at its highest level. The most important *biomarker* (a measurable indicator of some biological state or condition) of brain health that most people have never heard of is your rate of neurogenesis. *Neurogenesis* is the process of making new brain cells, the generation of new neurons. *Neurogenesis* is how the brain renews and upgrades itself.

Understanding neurogenesis is the most revolutionary discovery of neuroscience in the past century. Although there is still much to be learned, recent studies[1] have revealed that the process can be enhanced and encouraged by individual lifestyle choices. To increase neurogenesis is to improve your entire life—how you think, feel, and act.

Research shows that high rates of neurogenesis are associated with:

- higher cognitive function
- better memory and faster learning
- emotional vitality and resilience
- protection from stress, anxiety, and depression
- elevated immunity
- enhanced overall brain function

Increasing neurogenesis dramatically improves everyday life at all stages and radically transforms what aging looks and feels like.

Up until the late 1990s, neuroscience accepted as fact that the brain stops growing new brain cells by adulthood. It was believed that after this cessation, it was just one slow, unavoidable slide into decrepitude as brain cells die off, never to be replaced, gradually at first, but then faster and faster as you age. Then scientists discovered this was all wrong.

The discovery that your brain produces new brain cells as long as you are alive upends the belief that the brain stops growing in young adulthood. It also changes our entire picture of aging, for if new brain cells are being formed, then the brain can renew itself. What is key is the *rate* at which new brain cells form.

There are vast differences in how quickly people produce new brain cells, and your rate of neurogenesis may be the single most important factor for a high quality of life. When neurogenesis is high, you are alive, engaged, expansive, fulfilling your potential. Your mind's abilities are enhanced and your emotional vitality is strong. You are protected from stress and depression. You feel good and life is fulfilling. Immunity is robust. Your spirits are high and your outlook is positive.

With a low rate of neurogenesis, your brain shrinks, your life contracts, and you move toward memory loss, cognitive deficits, dementia, stress and anxiety, depression, reduced executive function, reduced immunity, and myriad health problems. When neurogenesis is low, your whole quality of life suffers. Having a high level of neurogenesis may be the most important thing you can do to cultivate a high quality of life.

We all hope for a simple solution—take this pill or eat this new food—and most self-help books offer relatively easy ways to change your life for the better. But this is not your typical self-help chapter. When it comes to the brain, almost nothing is simple. Given the brain's staggering complexity, a simple plan for brain health does not and cannot exist. It requires a multifaceted approach. We need to use our whole brain to enhance our whole brain.

Brain health is key to health in every area—physical, emotional, mental, spiritual. If present trends continue, 50 percent of adults aged eighty-five or older can expect to receive a diagnosis of Alzheimer's disease, which is marked by a dramatic loss of brain cells, especially in the hippocampus. Since most of the adult population today is expected to live longer than eighty-five, this means you have about a fifty-fifty chance of developing Alzheimer's. What's the point of keeping the body alive longer if you lose your mind?

Getting older doesn't have to be a downward spiral. Aging can mean getting wiser, deeper, more creative, more interesting and more interested, more joyful, more peaceful, more awake to the present moment, and evolving into a more loving human being. But for this to occur, you need to renew and enhance your brain's capacities, and this brings us to neurogenesis.

Holism understands we are complex beings that cannot be reduced to separate parts. The human organism operates as an integrated whole and can only be understood in the context of this wholeness. If a person loses a leg, it changes how the entire person balances and moves. If hearing is lost, the other senses increase to compensate. When someone is angry, it is expressed on physical, emotional, mental, and spiritual levels. Anything we do, think, see, or feel is experienced as an interrelated whole.

The only way to fully understand the brain is through a broad view that encompasses all of its possibilities for consciousness. Each level of body, heart, mind, and spirit has its own vibration or *energy frequency*, with the physical body being the densest and therefore having the lowest frequency.

Every level—physical, emotional, mental, spiritual—has its own "consciousness" that is experienced through the brain and contributes to the whole that is you. Only by considering and nurturing all four levels can the brain be fully understood and thus experience its highest development.

Purely physical or material approaches that try to understand the brain from the bottom up are woefully inadequate and leave out much that is essential. The majority of conventional neuroscience literature reduces the miracle of the human being to a cluster of neurotransmitters or biological processes divorced from relationships, beauty, and spirit.

Research data[2] show that providing an enriched environment stimulates the brain in multiple ways with a synergetic effect; that is, separate kinds of neurogenic activity—such as exercise, diet, emotional and cognitive stimulation—work together more powerfully than they do apart.

Different kinds of brain stimulation support each other. For instance, running boosts neurogenesis, but with running alone there is a 40–60 percent loss of these newly created brain cells. However, other parts of an enriched environment prevent neuronal cell loss but don't increase the number of new neurons formed. But put together, there is a large boost in new brain cells as well as an almost 100 percent survival rate. But only a holistic, multipronged approach produces the powerful boost in both new neurons and survival rates that result in a major increase in neurogenesis.

Currently, research in the Americas and Europe is overwhelmingly driven by financial concerns—pharmaceutical companies fund much of the research. Researchers looking to find the next big (selling) drug do much of the rest of the research; for example, it is possible to slightly tweak the molecular structure of a natural compound that has some biological effect so that this tweaked version can then be patented—regardless of its effectiveness. The lure of money distorts the research agenda to an appalling degree.

There are a few research centers, however, that are beginning to look at the bigger picture. One of these is the Buck Institute for Research on Aging in Novato, California. In the October 2014 issue of the journal *Aging,* researchers from the Buck Institute and UCLA reported the first known success for reversing Alzheimer's disease. Researchers using a simplified version of the strategy outlined in this chapter found greater success than had ever before been achieved.

Thus far, the prevailing wisdom has insisted that by the time Alzheimer's is noticed or diagnosed, there is so much damage to the brain that it's irreversible and unstoppable. Like someone falling down a cliff, nature must take its course, and the descent into increasing neural devastation is inevitable.

Indeed, billions have been invested to find a chemical compound that will stop or reverse the mental decline of Alzheimer's—with no success. Hundreds of clinical trials costing many billions of dollars have taken place, resulting only in failure after failure to even slow the disease's progression. Drugs have only had modest, temporary effects on symptoms. Nothing seemed to work.

Using a simplified version of this system described in this chapter, a pilot study found that memory loss may be reversed and the improvement sustained with this program. The study involved changing diet along some of the guidelines discussed here (such as eliminating sugar, reducing carbohydrates and processed food, and adding more vegetables and non-farmed salmon), plus adding just a few of the supplements discussed in this chapter, in conjunction with exercise, better sleep, and meditation.

Nine of the ten patients had a strong positive response to this program. Those who had left work due to memory problems or who were struggling at work were able to return to their employment with improved performance. These improvements have been sustained for two and a half years and counting after initial treatment.

Although this study was aimed at helping Alzheimer's patients, it included things that also happen to stimulate neurogenesis. Hopefully, this study is just the first step toward proving greater brain health can be achieved using the holistic strategy laid out here. In contrast, the *Neurogenesis* book focuses primarily upon increasing neurogenesis, with neurohealthy aging and Alzheimer's prevention as additional benefits.

My clinical practice with clients shows strong support for this approach. Using a neurogenesis-informed treatment strategy, I find my clients respond extremely well after just a few months. However, I have observed it takes a good year or two of following this program to create the most robust, rock-solid foundation in brain function and really feel the internal boost. Clients report feeling better than they've ever felt in their lives, with more energy and enthusiasm, more mental acuity and sharpness, and greater confidence than they believed possible.

"I've never felt so good in my life!" is a common remark. Such evidence is considered anecdotal, but it certainly shows where future research needs to go. The best evidence will come from your own observations when you compare your present experience to where you'll be in a year or two.

Diet and the Physical Level

The four most outstanding foods for stimulating neurogenesis are blueberries, omega-3 fatty acids, green tea, and curcumin.[4] It's worth considering making these a part of your regular diet.

Blueberries. It's hard to sing blueberries' praises highly enough. Blueberries act in so many ways to promote neurogenesis and protect the brain from cognitive decline that if blueberries were a drug, pharmaceutical companies would be bombarding us with ads to entice us to upgrade our brain with this "miracle drug."

Omega-3s. Another neurogenesis superstar is the complex of omega-3 fatty acids found in abundance in cold water fish, including wild Alaskan salmon, coho and sockeye salmon, black cod, sablefish, sardines, and herring. Omega-3s have been shown to dramatically increase neurogenesis and BDNF levels. (BDNF stands for Brain-Derived Neurotrophic Factor, which is like Miracle Grow for the brain, a peptide that increases neurogenesis and neural plasticity.) Neuroscience researcher Sandrine Thuret, PhD, of London's Kings College, reported a 40 percent increase in neurogenesis by adding omega-3s in *Science Daily* in 2007. Other studies[3] have shown equally impressive gains in neurogenesis, elevated BDNF levels, increased brain size, and neuroprotective benefits from omega-3s.

In the ongoing tearing down, replacing, and rebuilding of our brains' cellular structures, we want to consume high quality fats in order to continuously rebuild our brains with the best fats possible. Omega-3s *are* the highest quality fats for brain development. A diet high in unhealthy or "bad" fats slows down neurogenesis, but a diet high in healthy or "good" omega-3s increases neurogenesis to a higher level.

Green Tea. Green tea contains *polyphenols* (chemical compounds found in plants) the most powerful of which is *epigallocatechin gallate* (EGCG), a type of *catechin*. Green tea's polyphenols have been shown to increase neurogenesis, BDNF levels, and to have strong health benefits ranging from cancer prevention to fat loss, plus cardiovascular benefits, immunity improvement, and glucose reduction. ECGC and green tea's other polyphenols not only increase neurogenesis but also, like blueberries and omega-3s, have powerful antioxidant and anti-inflammatory effects as well. Green tea provides clear cognitive benefits and even improves working memory, which is one of the most difficult functions to increase.

Curcumin. Curcumin provides the yellow color in the curry spice turmeric. It has strong neurogenic effects. In addition, it is a powerful anti-inflammatory and antioxidant compound. Aging populations who consume curcumin show better cognitive performance. It reduces beta-amyloid and plaque formation in aging humans and has high potential as part of an anti-Alzheimer's strategy. It has also shown strong antidepressant effects, which naturally follow from decreasing inflammation and increasing neurogenesis.

The four foods above merit special attention for their neurogenesis- and brain health-promoting benefits, but there are numerous other nutrients that increase neurogenesis and BDNF levels. Since these often work via different metabolic pathways, eating a variety of foods that activate the brain from multiple directions is probably wiser than relying on a single source. *The Neurogenesis Diet and Lifestyle* discusses over thirty different nutrients that increase neurogenesis that most people would be wise to consider making part of their daily diet.

To recap the strategy: Diet and body practices to increase neurogenesis are step one in a holistic, four-fold plan to develop each part of our being: body, heart, mind, spirit. Equally important is stopping or avoiding things that shrink the brain and decrease neurogenesis and BDNF levels to ensure we don't erase the gains we make.

Two powerful ways of increasing neurogenesis are diet and aerobic exercise (other forms of exercise will not do, only aerobic exercise). Research on exercise is further along than research into nutrition, so more is known about the effects of exercise alone or exercise in combination with other factors. Exercise increases neurogenesis to four or five times its normal rate. However, only 40–60 percent of these new neurons survive. To boost these survival rates closer to 100 percent requires an enriched environment. The big question is: What does an "enriched environment" mean for humans?

We have some pretty good answers for this question, and they are integrated seamlessly into the holistic plan offered here in order to tease out the physical, emotional, mental, and spiritual dimensions to this question. First, let's look at the physical aspects of an enriched environment. These include:

- exercise (certain kinds)
- touch
- sexual experience
- sleep (7 or 8 hours per night)
- doing new things, being in novel environments, new sensory stimulation
- music, silence, natural sounds
- nature

The Emotional Level

The right kind of emotional stimulation leads to increased neurogenesis as well as emotional fulfillment. The wrong kind is neurotoxic and disrupts neurogenesis, even killing brain cells.

We tend to be unaware of how we spend our lives swimming in a sea of emotion. Neuroscience emphasizes how essential emotion is in organizing the brain and how key relationships are in this process.

Most people take their everyday relationships for granted, so much so that they tend to fade into the background like wallpaper. Yet these everyday relationships and how you feel throughout the day exert an immense effect upon your brain and neurogenesis.

The brain is wired for joy, love, interest, and excitement. It thrives in positive emotional conditions. Neurogenesis is ignited when you feel good. The brain functions at peak capacity when you feel your best.

The brain shrivels in the opposite conditions of stress, despair, lack of engagement, and depression. Neurogenesis and BDNF levels drop markedly. When you feel bad, your brain functions poorly.

The Mental Level

The human mind is the crown jewel of evolution. Science, art, culture, language, and a complex, well-developed self are some of the mind's highest attainments. The mind makes us human.

When we learn new things, the mind is stimulated and neurogenesis increases. By reading this chapter and learning about neurogenesis, you are increasing your rate of neurogenesis right now.

New learning is part of the "enriched environment" that allows recently created neurons to survive and thrive. For humans, an enriched environment consists of physical, emotional, mental, and spiritual stimulation. All are needed for the brain's full development. [2] But mental stimulation has a special place in this fourfold practice, for humanity is, in Aristotle's words, "the rational creature."

Actively engaging our minds pays off doubly: first, by promoting neurogenesis, and second, by enlarging our world. When we learn new things about our world, it expands our outlook and gives us a wider perspective on life.

Nowhere is the adage "use it or lose it" truer than with our minds. Cognitive testing shows there is a drop-off in mental abilities at two key points in life:

- after leaving school
- after retiring from work

Using our minds less is what both these key points have in common. When we slow down our mental engagement, we slow down our minds and neurogenesis. But note: Not everyone experiences such a decline. Those people who continue to be mentally engaged *do not* see a cognitive decline at these times.

Of course, we want to sharpen our mental abilities as much as possible and to stay sharp and alert for as long as possible. Research now shows that almost all cognitive decline is preventable. Some people in their nineties stay clear, focused, and sharp as a tack with no evidence of cognitive decline. Lifestyle factors greatly outweigh genetics in this. And while starting earlier in life is better than later, it's never too late to stimulate your mind, grow new neurons, and strengthen your cognitive capacities.

The Spiritual Level

Because of the materialistic bias in so much of science, very little research gets done on spirituality. Only recently have some neuroscientists investigated the effects of spiritual practices on the brain. What they've found isn't surprising to anyone who has a spiritual practice.

Although to a casual observer it may look like nothing is happening during meditation or prayer—just stillness and quiet sitting—on the inside the experience is powerfully dynamic and creative. This inner dynamism appears to strongly stimulate neurogenesis.

There are hundreds of types of spiritual practices among the many religions throughout the world. As research has developed, two key practices have been shown to help brain functioning. Since this field is just in its infancy, there will no doubt be others that future research reveals.

The two main practices that help brain function and appear to stimulate neurogenesis are mindfulness practices and devotion or compassion practices. Traditions of the Impersonal Divine focus on different approaches to mindfulness to discover the spiritual ground of our beings. Traditions of the Personal Divine focus on what can be called "heartfulness" practices of love, devotion, compassion, or surrender to discover our inmost souls.

It's important not to separate these practices too rigidly. In fact, both practices appear in both traditions, even though the emphasis differs in each. Thus, traditions of the Impersonal Divine that focus on mindfulness see compassion and loving kindness meditation as necessary preliminary practices, for we can only be as mindful as the heart is open. Similarly, traditions of the Personal Divine put their main emphasis upon devotional prayer and Bhakti meditation but see the calming of the mind (which can be brought about by mindfulness) as preparatory to opening the heart. Both practices appear to enhance neurogenesis.

Conclusion

As long as we are alive, the brain is renewing itself. Beginning environmental enrichment in middle age results in a fivefold increase in neurogenesis in old age. Thus far, there is little research on beginning an enriched environment in old age. Becoming more active by enhancing our brains' renewal in our seventies and eighties yields powerful results. Far better to do something and improve your life going forward than do nothing and decay more rapidly. Renewal is possible. The benefits of an "active life" for older adults are clear. Neurogenesis is always happening, and we can always increase its rate.

This is the path to continuous renewal: ongoing neurogenesis through actualizing our capacities and our self. We need to use our entire brains. Brain enhancement equals life enhancement.

References

1. Gage, F. (1998). "Neurogenesis in the adult human hippocampus" Nature Medicine. 4, 1313-1317

2. (Aug 2002) "Neuroplasticity in old age: Sustained fivefold induction of hippocampal neurogenesis by long-term environmental enrichment." Annals of Neurology. 52(2):135-43.

3. Beltz, B.S., Tlusty, M.F., Benton, J.L., Sandeman, D.C. (2007) "Omega-3 fatty acids upregulate adult neurogenesis," *Neuroscience Letters*.

4. Gage, F. (Aug 2000) "Reinventing the brain." *Life Extension Magazine* Interview.

5. Gomez-Pinilla, F. (2008). "Brain foods: The effects of nutrients on brain function" Nature Reviews Neuroscience. 9:568-578

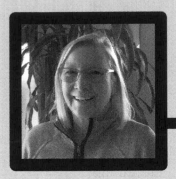

KATHLEEN K. FRY, MD, CTHHOM, ABIHM a past president of the American Holistic Medical Association (now the Academy of Integrative Health and Medicine) and a Founding Diplomate of the American Board of Integrative and Holistic Medicine, has trained in both conventional and holistic medicine, investing years of study to understand the true nature of healing.

She has incorporated homeopathy into her Ob/Gyn practice for over twenty-seven years. She works with clients of all kinds with a variety of health conditions and ailments to help them stimulate their body's ability to heal itself through the vibrational power of homeopathic medicine.

Her skill and expertise as a homeopathic physician have allowed her to help thousands of people discontinue pharmaceutical drugs and hormones and achieve the vibrant health that is our birthright.

Dr. Fry is the author of two books: *VITALITY! How to Get It and Keep It: A Homeopath's Guide to Vibrant Health without Drugs* (Amazon.com) *and What's the Remedy for That? The Definitive Homeopathy Guide to Mastering Everyday Self-Care without Drugs.* She speaks to both professional and lay groups about homeopathy and holistic health for men, women, and children. She is available for private consultations via telephone, Skype, or by arrangement from Boulder, Colorado.

www.drkathifry.com
drkathi@drkathifry.com
kathleen.fry 180 via Skype

CHAPTER 13

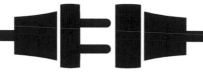

How to Have Vibrant Health and Vitality at Any Age *without* Drugs—A Homeopathy Primer for Seniors

By **KATHLEEN K. FRY, MD**

I t's a common misconception that it is normal to become tired and worn out as we age. How many times have you been told (or maybe even told yourself) that "it's just your age?" As a physician with more than thirty years' experience caring for people of all ages, I have heard this comment innumerable times. But I have also cared for people well into their eighties who run circles around their peers and seem to have boundless energy. What's their secret? Is it just good genes? Have they found the perfect combination of vitamins? What is it that gives them so much energy that they really do seem to run like the Energizer Bunny?

I discovered this "secret" more than twenty-five years ago when I became sick myself. I had been practicing medicine for about sixteen years when I developed a severe case of insomnia due to stress and overwork. I was exhausted but I could not sleep to save my life. I could barely get through a day of surgery and seeing an office full of patients. I began to suffer from low-grade headaches because my blood pressure was very high.

Fortunately, I had begun studying homeopathic medicine several years before, and I knew that there was a safe and effective alternative to taking prescription drugs. I consulted with a homeopath who recommended a remedy for me. After the first dose, I slept like a baby for the first time in weeks. As I continued to take the remedy, my blood pressure returned to normal, and I never had to take any prescription medications.

Just like my Energizer Bunny patients, I have all the energy I need to get through a full, busy day. And I have not taken a prescription medication in almost thirty years, quite a feat for a medical doctor with a prescription pad!

What I learned from my own experience and that of many of my patients is the key to understanding the source of vitality and good health. Homeopathic medicine not only explains how we get sick; it also holds the key to regaining our health and vitality without relying on pharmaceutical drugs. And that's the information I want to share with you if you're interested in having vibrant health without having to take a handful of pills several times a day.

The Spiritual Vital Force

This state of vibrant emotional, mental, and physical health is possible no matter how many birthdays you have had. Not only is it possible, it is also absolutely necessary in order for you to fulfill your soul's true purpose.

We are spirit beings inhabiting "skin suits," our bodies. The body does not run itself. It is controlled by an unseen power that Dr. Samuel Hahnemann, the father of homeopathy, termed the "Vital Force": the "spirit-like *dynamis* that rules the body with unbounded sway." It is the force that traditional Chinese physicians call *chi* and the Ayurvedic physicians of India call *prana*.

What does this mean in our daily lives? Every second of every minute of every hour of every day, our bodies perform many, many functions without our conscious control. Imagine if you *consciously* had to direct your body to make bone marrow, digest breakfast, and grow hair and toenails every day—you would have no time to use a computer, read a book, take a walk, or even just take out the trash.

All of the wondrous things that our bodies do without our conscious input are under the control of the Vital Force. But unlike functions of the body that can be measured with blood tests, evaluated with CT scans, or examined by doctors, the Vital Force is *unseen*. It is only by observing its *effects* that we are able to assess its strength.

You can feel when your own Vital Force is strong and when it is weak. When it is strong, you awaken refreshed after a night of deep, satisfying, *unmedicated* sleep. You get out of bed easily without pain in your back or your joints, and you can start your day *without needing any pills.* When the Vital Force is strong and healthy, you don't have to take medications or other substances to wake up. *You are already* awake, alive, and ready to go.

When you have a strong Vital Force, you feel balanced emotionally and have a reservoir of patience that allows you to be kind and loving with your family members, friends, colleagues, and even casual acquaintances. You've probably experienced just the opposite condition at times in your life.

When the Vital Force is weak and unhealthy, you can't sleep well. You toss and turn or wake up in the middle of the night and can't go back to sleep unless you take a pill—and even that doesn't always work. When you lack essential vitality, you have stiff joints or aching muscles and wish you could just stay in bed. You feel cranky, irritable, and sometimes quite *angry* about how you feel. So your family members walk around "on eggshells" because they've learned that if they cross you, there will be hell to pay.

When you feel this exhausted, your sex drive is gone. Without vitality, you don't have the emotional stamina to support those who rely on you for strength: your family, your friends, and your coworkers.

Without a well-functioning Vital Force, you cannot fulfill your soul's purpose. What does this mean? It means that each of us is born, as the Bible says, in the image of the Creator. You are born to create and to re-create. You are born to fulfill your soul's destiny. Your task as a human is to learn what that destiny is and to attain it. You have been given certain skills and talents, and if you pay attention to and follow the guidance of your heart, you will discover what it is that you were born to do.

Michael Jordan was not born to be a fireman or a world-famous chef, and certainly not a curveball-hitting outfielder for the Chicago White Sox. By following his passion for basketball, he developed his innate talents to become the greatest athlete of his time. And that required *vitality* in addition to vision, drive, and commitment. If, God forbid, he had been born sickly, or his parents had failed to feed him properly, we would never have known his name.

It is not enough to be born with talent. That talent needs to be discovered, nurtured, and developed. And when that happens, mastery and magic occur. You have your own set of innate abilities, the mastery of which contributes to the betterment of the world. You don't have to be a Michael Jordan to make a big difference in your own life and the lives of those you love. But you *must* have the vitality and stamina to do what you need to do.

The Vital Force, or Spirit, follows certain universal laws or principles. Although we cannot see, touch, taste, hear, or smell them, we can and do observe the effects of these principles on our lives each day. The Vital Force governs every cell of our beings. It is that unseen Force that tells our cells to divide in two instead of three, or four, or seven. It is what guides the sperm to find the egg and begin the process of creating an entire human being "from scratch." It is what gives us the patience to read *Good Night, Moon* to our grandkids over and over again, night after night after night.

This powerful Vital Force is responsible for maintaining good, vibrant health. When the Vital Force is weakened, it communicates its need for help by giving us symptoms. Those symptoms are the "language" of the Vital Force. Understanding that language and how to give the Vital Force what it needs forms the basis for healing through the art and science of homeopathic medicine.

What Is Homeopathy?

Homeopathy is a form of healing that uses natural substances prepared in a special way in a homeopathic pharmacy to strengthen the spiritual Vital Force and restore us to health.

Homeopathy comes from the Greek words "homeos," meaning similar, and "pathos," meaning suffering. Homeopathic medicines work on the principle that *like heals like*: A substance that brings on a set of symptoms when given to a healthy person can be used to strengthen the Vital Force in a sick person exhibiting those same symptoms. As the spiritual Vital Force is restored, the symptoms diminish and eventually disappear.

The power of homeopathic remedies is revealed when volunteers take them in a process known as a *proving*. For example, in the proving of Arsenicum album, Dr. Hahnemann tested this substance on healthy volunteers by giving them a 3c potency of a mother tincture of arsenic. A mother tincture is made by dissolving arsenic in alcohol. The 3c potency of arsenic is made by taking one drop of the mother tincture and serially diluting it in 99 drops of water 3 times. Once the desired potency is achieved, in this case the 3c, the liquid is poured on milk sugar pellets. The healthy volunteers are given one pellet daily until they begin to develop symptoms.

In the proving of arsenic, the volunteers developed nausea, vomiting, abdominal cramps, and chills. These are the hallmark symptoms of food poisoning. In this way, Hahnemann discovered that a homeopathic preparation of arsenic, called Arsenicum album, could be used to treat food poisoning. The information gathered in the proving of a large number of natural substances is recorded in what is known as the *Materia Medica*. This body of knowledge allows a homeopath to choose from more than five thousand remedies in order to annihilate disease and restore vibrant health.

The History of Homeopathy

How did homeopathy come about? This is one of the most fascinating yet widely unknown stories in the history of Western medicine. Dr. Samuel Hahnemann (1755-1843) was a physician who lived and worked in Germany, primarily in Saxony. He was appalled by the techniques that passed for healing treatments by the doctors of his time. In those days, disease was thought to be due to an imbalance of the four "humors": black bile (*melanchole*), yellow bile (*chole*), phlegm (*phlegma*), and blood (*sanguis*). This theory had been the basis of medical practice since the time of Hippocrates.

Treatments were designed to restore the balance of these humors by such drastic means as sweating, purging, vomiting, and bloodletting. Toxic substances such as arsenic and mercury were used to treat diseases such as syphilis, which was rampant throughout Europe in the eighteenth century.

Hahnemann saw that the treatments were often worse than the disease they were attempting to eliminate. So he quit the practice of medicine. But he had a wife and seven children to feed, so he supported his family by translating into German ancient medical texts written in Greek and Latin by such luminaries as Hippocrates, Galen, and Paracelsus. During this time of intensive study, Hahnemann realized a deep truth that would lead to a radical new system of healing.

In the "Introduction" to the *Organon of Medicine*, 6th edition, Hahnemann explains:

"As long as men have existed, they have been liable, individually or collectively, to diseases from physical or moral causes. In a rude state of nature but few remedial agents were required, as the simple mode of living admitted of but few diseases; with the civilization of mankind in the state, on the contrary, the occasions of diseases and the necessity for medical aid increased in equal proportion. But ever since that time (soon after Hippocrates, therefore, for 2500 years) men have occupied themselves with the treatment of (an) ever-increasing multiplicity of diseases, who led astray by their vanity, sought by reasoning and guessing to excogitate the mode of furnishing this aid. *Innumerable and dissimilar ideas* respecting the nature of diseases and their remedies sprang from so many dissimilar brains, and the theoretical views these gave rise to the so-called systems, each of which was at variance with the rest and self-contradictory" (italics added).

In other words, the medical practices and procedures used in Hahnemann's day were based not on objective findings but on numerous random theories put forth and debated among various schools of medical thought. This continued to be true in Hahnemann's time when there was no innate understanding of how the body healed or what caused people to be sick. New treatments were being introduced arbitrarily based on nothing but conjecture and speculation.

An unexpected development occurred about the same time that led Hahnemann to create an entirely new system of healing and to return to caring for patients. In 1790, Hahnemann was translating a medical paper from English into German written by William

Cullen, a Scottish physician. Dr. Cullen maintained that Peruvian *cinchona* (quinine) bark was effective for treating malaria because of its tonic effect on the stomach. Hahnemann was unconvinced of this because there were many so-called stomach tonics that were not effective in treating malaria.

Dr. Hahnemann decided to experiment on himself and proceeded to take small amounts of quinine bark for several days. What do you suppose happened? If you guessed that he developed the symptoms of malaria, you would be right. Mind you, the malarial parasite wasn't identified until nearly a century later.

In Hahnemann's time, no one knew about the association between malaria and mosquitoes. Without being bitten by a parasite-carrying mosquito, Hahnemann developed a full-blown case of malaria with its distinctly characteristic fever alternating with chills and delirium. How could this happen? By taking this substance, Hahnemann demonstrated the Law of Similars. Everything that God created has both an energetic as well as a physical component. When someone gets bitten by a mosquito bearing the parasite that causes malaria, there is an energy that is transmitted to a person's Vital Force from the parasite. The Vital Force responds by producing distinct symptoms: shaking chills, alternating with fever. When a healthy volunteer takes a diluted form of quinine, it brings on the same symptoms as someone infected by the mosquito. Giving the infected person a homeopathic preparation of quinine, stimulates the person's Vital Force to "rev up" their immune system and combat the parasitic infection.

This extraordinary development was actually the first proving of a homeopathic remedy. Hahnemann kept meticulous notes about his symptoms, including the subjects of his dreams, the foods he craved, his moods, and his thinking patterns.

This record became the first entry in the homeopathic *Materia Medica* [2], and the remedy today is known as *china officinalis*. Not only does it successfully restore the Vital Force of a person with symptoms of malaria, it is also a very effective remedy for weakness brought on by loss of bodily fluids. It is one of our most important remedies for hemorrhage after childbirth and the subsequent anemia that results.

Once Hahnemann discovered the power of the proving process, he began to test other substances, including the most commonly prescribed medicines of his day, arsenic and mercury. Hahnemann catalogued the underlying principles of homeopathy in a book called the *Organon of Medicine*. In the very first paragraph of this work, Hahnemann clearly stated the *raison d'etre* for every physician: "The physician's high and only mission is to restore the sick to health, to cure, as it is termed."

Notice that Hahnemann did *not* say: "The physician's high and only mission is to keep people on many medications for their entire lives, with continued decline in their health." In fact, Hahnemann said just the *opposite (Organon,* 6th edition, paragraph 9):

"In the healthy condition of man, the spiritual Vital Force (autocracy), the dynamis that animates the material body (organism) rules with unbounded sway, and retains all the parts of the organism in admirable, harmonious, vital operation, as regards both sensations and functions, so that our indwelling, reason-gifted mind can freely employ this living, healthy instrument for the higher purposes of our existence." [1]

In other words, the Vital Force or what Hahnemann called the "spirit like dynamis" is the unseen force that is responsible for maintaining living beings in a state of healthy homeostasis. Being in this healthy state allows us to fulfill our purpose in life.

When that homeostasis is disrupted by an outside force (a parasite, a bacterium, emotional trauma, etc.) the Vital Force "asks" for the assistance it needs by producing a specific symptom picture. A trained homeopath recognizes that symptom picture from the provings of the substance done on healthy volunteers.

That is how we know which homeopathic remedy to prescribe for which condition.

Homeopathic Remedies for Seniors

While homeopathy is an individualized form of medicine, there are remedies that can be used for acute conditions that are readily available in most health food stores. Here is a list of remedies used for common ailments. As a general rule, take the 30 c potency by mouth. The number of pellets doesn't matter because the pellets are just a carrier for the healing energy. Also as a general rule, you should not eat, drink, or brush your teeth twenty minutes before or after taking a remedy to allow it to work.

In acute situations where the symptoms are severe, you can repeat the remedy every three to four hours. As the symptoms subside, cut back on the frequency and take the remedy two or three times a day until all your symptoms are gone. Then take the remedy once a day for three days after you are symptom-free; this prevents a relapse.

Aconitum napellus: Also known as *Aconite*, this remedy is indicated for a cold that comes on suddenly, usually after exposure to cold, windy weather. Symptoms usually include a headache, sore throat, and a cough. The key indication for using this remedy is the *sudden* onset of illness. It's also the first remedy to take in cases of *shock* of any kind (emotional, mental, or physical).

Arnica montana: This is the classic remedy to take for *injury* or *trauma*. When taken right away, it prevents bruising and reduces pain. It's the perfect remedy to take *after a fall* or after surgery. If the injury is severe, take the 200 c potency instead of the 30 c. Most health food stores carry the 200 c.

Arsenicum album: Nausea, vomiting, stomach cramps, and anxiety about being so ill are the classic symptoms calling for this powerful remedy for *food poisoning*. (I have personally used this remedy for food poisoning on four separate vacations and never had to take antibiotics or go to the hospital.) The key is to take the 30 c potency every 15-30 minutes as soon as the symptoms start. Initially, the symptoms will worsen as your body purges the energy that came in on the contaminated food. As your symptoms lessen, take the remedy hourly, then every few hours. Continue the remedy two or three times a day until you are well; then take it once a day for three more days to prevent a recurrence. If you feel weak or can't keep fluids down, see a doctor right away; you may need IV fluids. However, in most cases, if you start the remedy right away, you can avoid getting dehydrated.

Bryonia alba: Pain or any other complaint that is made worse with motion calls for *Bryonia alba*. Arthritis pain, and any pain from pneumonia, colds, and the flu that become worse when moving around call for this remedy.

Cocculus indicus: This is a classic remedy for caregivers who are *exhausted from nursing the sick*. Feeling tired from worry and lack of sleep are common symptoms calling for this remedy. Take the 30 c potency at bedtime and again in the morning. You can continue it twice a day until you feel well again, and then slowly wean off the remedy, taking it less frequently over the course of a week.

Coffea cruda: Made from raw, green coffee beans, this remedy is very helpful for *insomnia* due to an overactive mind. These are the classic symptoms elucidated in the proving of Coffea cruda done on healthy volunteers. When you're lying in bed and you can't get to sleep because your brain just won't quiet down, a 30 c of this remedy usually does the trick. You can take another dose if you awaken during the night and can't get back to sleep. The advantage to taking homeopathic remedies instead of sleeping pills is there are no side effects, such as sleepwalking or morning drowsiness.

Ferrum phosphoricum: Unlike *Aconite*, which is indicated for a cold that comes on suddenly, this remedy is the one to take at the first sign of a sore throat, runny nose, or a cough that comes on gradually. Taking the 30 c every four hours can often shorten the course of a cold and lessen the severity of the symptoms.

Gelsemium sempervirens: Body aches, headache, and profound weakness due to *flu* call for this remedy. Taking the 30 c potency every 2-3 hours works better than Tamiflu or over-the-counter drugs in cases of flu. Taking this remedy often helps prevent the chronic fatigue that can linger after a bad case of flu.

Nux vomica: This is a great remedy for *heartburn* and *stomach upset* that are commonly diagnosed as gastroesophageal reflux, or GERD. It's cheaper and more effective than the "purple pill" and has no side effects. It's also a great remedy for a hangover or stomach upset from overeating spicy food.

Podophyllum peltatum: This remedy works wonders for travelers who develop diarrhea from eating tainted food. Green- or yellowish-colored stool that comes out "in a gush" calls for this remedy. You can take the 30 c hourly until it stops.

Rhus toxicodendron (tox): This remedy is a lifesaver for those who suffer with arthritis pain that has very particular symptoms. People who need *Rhus tox* complain that they are very stiff in the morning; they feel a bit better once they get up and start moving around. However, if they overdo it by exercising too much or walking too far, the stiffness returns. Taking this remedy in the 30 c potency at bedtime and again in the morning can bring relief from pain that can seem miraculous. For those who have suffered with arthritis for many years, it's best to see a homeopathic practitioner for guidance on how to adjust the potency over time. The 30 c potency may bring immediate relief, but for those with chronic pain, they will most likely need higher potencies of *Rhus tox* for longer periods of time to bring permanent relief.

Staphysagria: Made from the flower *Delphinium*, this is the "go to" remedy for a bladder infection, especially if it occurs after a catheter is inserted into the bladder. Symptoms include painful, frequent urination with blood in the urine. Take the 30 c potency every 3-4 hours to relieve the symptoms. Continue the remedy until the urine tests clear. You can get a urine test kit in the pharmacy that will tell you when the infection has cleared. It often takes longer to clear the urine than it would if you were using antibiotics, but there are no side effects, and the infection is less likely to recur when treated homeopathically.

Lastly, if you enjoy traveling, these three remedies are especially helpful for *jet lag*: *Arnica* for muscle stiffness, *Cocculus indicus* for sleep disruption, and *Nux vomica* for stomach upset. You can take all three remedies together every few hours at the start of a trip and arrive refreshed at your destination.

Homeopathic medicines are safe, effective, and very inexpensive; a tube containing eighty-five doses of a wide variety of remedies is readily available in most natural food stores for less than $10.00. These remedies can be used, for example, to treat allergies without using over-the-counter medicines that commonly have side effects and don't cure the underlying problem, which is a weakness in the Vital Force that manifests as sensitivity to blooming plants.

Similarly, there are remedies to treat infections without antibiotics, to restore thyroid function without thyroid hormone, and to relieve menopausal symptoms without hormone therapy. You can learn how to use these over-the-counter remedies when you have a cold or the flu and save yourself an expensive trip to the doctor or the emergency room.

I'd like to share an experience I had myself where homeopathy saved me a visit to the emergency room while I was on a ski vacation. I was headed to Utah, and I had a sandwich at the Denver airport just before boarding my flight. I have not taken a prescription drug in almost thirty years; instead, I rely solely on homeopathic medicine. As a result, my Vital Force is exquisitely tuned, and I react immediately whenever I encounter what Dr. Hahnemann called "a morbific influence inimical to life." Within twenty minutes of finishing my lunch, I began to feel light-headed and queasy. By the time we were airborne, I had all the symptoms of food poisoning: nausea, vomiting, abdominal cramps, and a bad case of chills. Fortunately, I never travel without *Arsenicum album*, the most common remedy for food poisoning. As its name implies, it is made from arsenic diluted in one hundred drops of water thirty times. I took the 30 c potency every fifteen minutes because my symptoms were so severe. As my symptoms started to lessen, I took the remedy less frequently. By the time I got to the resort, I was taking the remedy every two hours. I went to sleep for a few hours and when I awoke, I was completely well. I slept like a baby, ate a big breakfast the next morning, and enjoyed three full days of skiing without any hint of illness. I continued to take the remedy once a day for the next few days to be sure my Vital Force completely annihilated the tainted energy that had attached itself to my lunch.

This is the power of homeopathy, and I am on a mission to educate people on the safe and effective use of these remedies. To that end, I have written a new book called, *What's the Remedy for That? The Definitive Homeopathy Guide to Mastering Everyday Self-Care without Drugs*. You can get a copy from Amazon.com, or you can ask your local bookstore to order a copy for you from the publisher, IngramSpark.

I hope you find this information helpful and I encourage you to try a homeopathic remedy the next time you have a cold or the flu. The art and science of homeopathy can be your path to vibrant health *at any age* without having to rely on pharmaceutical drugs.

References

1. Organon of Medicine, Samuel Hahnemann, MD, 6th Editon, translated by William Boericke, MD, reprint edition, 1993, B. Jain Publishers Pvt, Ltd, New Delhi, India.

2. *Materia Medica Pura* Hahnemann, Samuel; Arnoldischen Buchhandlung, Dresden. Germany: 1811-1821

A Final Word

Aging *is* definitely a challenge, however, it is also an opportunity and a privilege. *We are the lucky ones.* Just look at all of the people that you have known who have not made it this far along the path of life.

You and I are still here, and can choose to enjoy life, continue to learn, and leave a legacy. The other day, I mentioned to my four-year-old grandson, Calvin, that he was growing up so fast that it was getting harder to get him into his car seat. He smiled and said that when he was an adult, he would miss me because I would probably be dead—-then he stopped and said, "I mean in heaven." I asked him why he thought I would be gone, and he said because I was getting older. Then I asked, "Well how old do you think I am?" He stopped, looked as if he was sizing me up, and after a few moments said, "Twenty-eight." I started laughing, and told him that he was close, but that I thought I would be around for a while. By the way, I am sixty-seven and his mom is thirty-eight.

My goal is to be able to enjoy life to the fullest regardless of age. I also wish the same for you. That is why I created this book. All of my contributors are not only experts in their fields, but also passionate about helping others. They are also incredible presenters and speakers who can motivate audiences to take charge of their health and lives. I invite you to check out their websites, books and services.

So what is the take-a-way from this book? Here it is: "Make the rest of your life the BEST of your life." This is your time to finally slow down and decide what it is that YOU WANT to do instead of what you HAVE to do. If you have the proper mind set, take good care of your body, and have a great support team, your chances of success are excellent! How amazing would it be to be so *distracted* by enjoying life that you never even realize that you are getting older? That's what Empowered Aging is all about!

Best to YOU!

Sharkie Zartman